LETTERS TO YOUNG IOWAN

Good Sense From
The Good Folks of Iowa
For Young People Everywhere

Edited by
Zachary Michael Jack

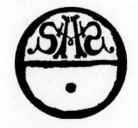

Ice Cube Press
North Liberty, Iowa

Letters To A Young Iowa:
Good Sense from the Good Folks of Iowa
For Young People Everywhere

Copyright © 2007 Ice Cube Press
Marvin Bell's letter copyright © 2007 by Marvin Bell

Isbn 1-888160-21-7 (9781888160215)

Library of Congress Control Number: 2006936413

Ice Cube Press (est. 1993)
205 North Front Street
North Liberty, Iowa 52317-9302
www.icecubepress.com
steve@icecubepress.com

Manufactured in the United States of America.

∞ The paper used in this publication meets the minimum requirements of
the American National Standard for Information Sciences—Permanence
of Paper for Printed Library Materials, ANSI Z39.48-1992

Mary Swander's, "A Home-Grown Solution for Iowa, Slow-Food Movement Creates Healthy Future," appeared in the Des Moines Register, July 9,
2006.

Cover art by Shelly Maxwell © 2007

For you, young Iowan,
and for all your dreams

TABLE OF CONTENTS

A Foreword by Governor Robert D. Ray

Iowa native Zachary Michael Jack, the editor of *Letters to a Young Iowan*, has provided a compilation of meaningful communications from experienced, successful Iowa leaders and everyday citizens—messages that, if taken seriously, can have a profound effect on readers.

The other day I followed a young man through the airport who was wearing a gray T-shirt that said *It's all about attitude*. I couldn't agree more. Attitude is a choice, and people who choose a positive attitude are happy people. Happiness is the foundation for accomplishment and success.

Life is challenging but also very rewarding. Life is chock-full of opportunities that mean little unless seized. Life can be discouraging, yet, depending on one's attitude, it can also be exciting and encouraging.

As one outgrows childhood, one realizes that happiness is dependent on character—making good choices and doing the right thing. What you do reflects on who you are. The essential elements of good character are trustworthiness, respect, responsibility, fairness, caring, and citizenship. These are the Six Pillars of Character. They are practiced in Iowa through an initiative I helped lead called Character Counts.

The letters in *Letters to a Young Iowan* are written by older Iowans—many famous, others on their way to fame, and still others who would rather not be famous at all—to younger Iowans. They are all about gratitude and character. Like our Character Counts initiative, they reach out to Iowa's young people where they live and do so with the power to transform. But it's a two-way street. The students to whom these letters are written are just half the audience. The other half are seasoned Iowans, those of us who write letters to young people, whether children, grandchildren, nieces, nephews, or former students or athletes we helped mentor. In reading our own letters and the letters of others, we remember our shared beliefs. In the quiet space offered by a letter, we reflect on our own character.

Over the decades, especially during my years as Iowa's Governor, I received thousands of letters. Many were thank-you notes. I treasured those notes

Good Sense from the Good Folks of Iowa

because each contained an expression of appreciation; someone sat down and took the time to convey a message just to me. Also, I recall vividly letters I received when I was overseas in military service. They connected me with my family back home and kept me in touch—a memory I'll have all my life.

These letters from a who's who of contemporary Iowans provide a similar pleasure. They reach out across space and time, reminding all of us who we are and where home is. They remind us that no matter how far away from Iowa we roam or how difficult our lives become, Iowa will always be there for us, quietly teaching and giving. Such letters are not only a way to communicate, inform, preserve information, and stay in touch, they can provide comfort.

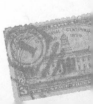

ACKNOWLEDGMENTS

This book would not have been possible without the goodwill, good hearts, and good vibes of its many contributors. To them, I am deeply indebted, and, before them, I am deeply humbled. Among them, Jim Autry, Tom Dean, Roger Farmer, Mary Swander and Timothy Walch deserve special recognition for their timely referrals and abiding interest. Gary Grant and Kitty Olsen were instrumental in facilitating contributions from Representative Jim Leach and Governor Robert D. Ray, who likewise have my utmost appreciation. Duane Acker, Marvin Bell, Scott Cawelti, Dan Gable, Neil Harl, Barbara Lounsberry, Myrna Sandvik, Robert Sayre, and the other emeritus, retired, or distinguished professors and coaches in this collection merit special recognition for their many years of service to Iowa's young people. For bringing you the voices of these distinguished Iowans, Steve Semken has my profound gratitude.

Personally, I would be remiss not to thank Kris Clark, Brion Hurley, Jeff Kaufmann, Neil Nakadate, Rodney Sullivan, and Kevin Woods for standing by a friend and colleague and his pie-eyed passions. And to my family, I owe everything.

Editor's Introduction:
Winter, Spring, Summer or Fall,
All You Got to Do Is Call: A Year of
Letters to a Young Iowan

Zachary Michael Jack

I dropped the question one night at our family supper on the farm, the dinner table always the best spot for news of pregnancies, comings out, worries about health.

What's the single most important piece of advice you would give a young Iowan?

You might have heard a pin drop. Silence, then the slowly building sounds of an ecstatic, Iowa family feed starting up again, undaunted, like so many cicadas, like a spooked cricket tentatively finding its tune again, taking it from the top. The groaning, sighing, slurping, and all around masticating recommenced and, when the family came up for breath, they rehashed, *Single most important piece of advice …? That's easy*, they said.

Leave.

They were kidding, naturally.

Only a family like ours, happily ensconced on the same Iowa farm for over one hundred and fifty years, could indulge such loose and ironic talk. And don't think we haven't had our chances in the past century-and-a-half for a fling with the Sun Belt or a dalliance with the Delta. We've been to the crossroads.

Take my grandparents, for instance. Like so many Iowa farm folks, they snowbirded their brood down to Florida a week or two each winter in the 1950s, always staying at the same Ma 'n Pa hotel in Naples and always getting morose when it came time to come home. When one year Ma 'n Pa up and offered to sell the whole shebang to my grandfolks, the devil danced a jig by Florida moonlight, eager to test his Tempter's mettle against the two most difficult existential eggs to crack: a seed corn salesman and his wife. *Do you want to suffer through January in Iowa your whole damn life, Edward,* Beelzebub demanded of my grandfather, *scooping snow, having the snot freeze on your nose?* (The devil speaks more crudely than this, you understand ... but modesty prevents me.) To my grandmother he said, *And you, Julia, how you long to collect conch shells and pastel parasols, not walnuts and sorrows.* Sounding like a realtor, he continued, *Naples is Florida's little city with the big, big future! Know Naples,* he said, insinuating the city slogan and its impressive vitals—*76 mild degrees year-round, population 6,500 to 8,500.* The devil winked ironically when next he hissed the Florida State Motto: *In God We Trust.*

So, yea, we have traveled through the vale of darkness, and yea, we have seen the light.

❧❧

It was February and the letters to young Iowans, like the weather, were erratic. Most days I'd tromp to the mailbox to touch nothing but junk mail or cold steel. More often I'd pour myself a cup of tea, flick on the computer, and wait while the cyber elves ventured into the cool, silicon blue to retrieve what letters to a young Iowan might have arrived by e-mail overnight. Well into March, the elves came back mostly empty-handed, surly and bickering among themselves.

But as the weather warmed and the trees greened, the letters, and especially the e-mails, started to trickle in. Slowly, I began to look forward to checking the mailbox each day, offering the cyber elves a cup of Earl Grey while they regaled me with news of their travels, as I in my slippers—I in my cap—settled down to appraise the day's catch.

The letters hadn't arrived by accident. I had spent the better part of several months sending out invites by the dozens, hundreds in all, to every seasoned Iowan I could think of worthy of inclusion. Still more calls for submissions were doled out by hand at in-state conferences and posted to Iowa newspapers and listservs. Sadly, some invitees never responded. Others said they would be glad to write a letter under other circumstances ... they were sorry but they were just too busy. Was this still the Iowa I knew as a boy, I wondered, the state of slow walks and languid porch swings,

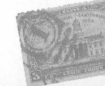

the state of *we'll-make-time?* Many of my invitations, I was convinced, lay whimpering, unattended, in drafty cyber inboxes around the state. I started thinking fatalistically, like an actuary or a slumping big leaguer about to get sent down to the minors—*Let's see if I average a response rate of ten percent … that means to get thirty letters I would need to send out a total of …*

As I prepared to order the flowers for the funeral of *Letters to a Young Iowan*, I resolved, in its final moments, to work the phones like a madman, like a Kennedy hell-bent on electing Jack. In one moment of desperation-induced courage, I called Dan Gable. I was rehearsing a pathetic, self-pitying voicemail when the legend picked-up, gruff like a family doc woken up in the wee hours. It will surprise no one who knows Dan Gable's generosity, his heart, and his commitment to the state that he was able to look past my tongue-tied, awestruck disaster-of-an-invite. Not so many weeks later, his letter arrived. I kissed it like a war bride.

A.D. (After Dan), a groundswell started happening; the monkey was off my back. Potential contributors wrote to say something was brewing, and that if an hour or two could be set aside here or there, well, who knows? Whom should they picture as their audience, they wondered, just in case? To whom should they write? Many envisioned a grandson or granddaughter, others a student, and still others an amalgam of what demographers, pollsters, and politicos say constitutes Iowa youth. Mentally, they collaged a composite image from bits and bobs of old magazines and newspapers, from snaps and snails and puppy dog tails and all things nice. *Make it intimate*, I said. *Write as you would talk. But also make it universal, so that no matter what young Iowan you're writing, I'll feel like you're writing to me.*

If you build it they will come, I might have said.

Late in April the collection received a boost, in spirit at least, from the passage of the Iowa Studies Bill, SF 2320, directing the Department of Cultural Affairs to assist Iowa teachers in finding ways to incorporate Iowa studies into their classrooms. The zeitgeist, I convinced myself, had turned in favor of Iowa as a subject worthy of study. I began to reconsider *Letters* as a potential textbook for a *living* history of Iowa, a cultural and historical primer for what we are, what we've been, and especially where we're going—

what the poet William Butler Yeats described as "what is past, passing, or to come."

With SF 2320 on the books, it seemed an ideal time to ask the historians among the contributors to write a famous or infamous historical Iowan. These writers, juggling the difficult intimacies of a letter with the vagaries of history, faced a double challenge. But the historians rose to the challenge, as they always do, crafting instructive, time-traveling dispatches to such famous Iowans as wrestling legend Frank Gotch, Herbert Hoover, Glenn Miller, Henry A. Wallace, Laura Ingalls Wilder, and, of course, Grant Wood.

To be a letter-coach, as I suddenly found myself, gave me a chance to dust off my big-brother/uncle skills. It gave me a chance, quite literally, to be *avuncular*. In corresponding with a growing number of letter writers, I coaxed, I pleaded, I encouraged, I affirmed. I read, re-read, and revised drafts by the dozens, sending proposed edits back to the writers for their stamp of approval or for further fiddling. Sometimes I cracked the whip so loud the cyber elves went running. Other times I went all warm and fuzzy. By May, a few letters a week were showing up, slow and steady like a good spring rain. It occurred to me, belatedly, that to solicit, compile, and edit a collection of letters, from scratch, meant that I, too, would need to live and breathe epistles. I had become, to my horror and bemusement, a letter-jockey.

About this time I began filling a library copy of the German poet Ranier Maria Rilke's book *Letters to a Young Poet* with that special brand of hyper-light pencil mark you can erase before turning a borrowed book back in, fine-free. When my conscience got the better of me (in a former life I had worked as a public librarian in Ames), I switched to lizard-green, iridescent sticky notes to mark the many memorable passages I was encountering. *Seek the depth of things*, the great poet wrote his young friend, the college student Franz Cappus; *there Irony never descends*. The two had struck up an unlikely conversation, the twenty-year-old Cappus—who was attending a military academy in Germany in the autumn of 1902 and who feared he might be becoming a poet—and Rilke, the great man of letters. "And without having intended to do so at all," Cappus remembers, "I found myself writing a cover letter in which I unreservedly laid bare my heart as never before and

never since to any second human being." Unbelievably, Rilke's reply arrived not so many weeks later in a blue, sealed envelope postmarked Paris. The letters would keep coming until 1908, when, Cappus later recalled, they "petered out because life drove me off into those very regions from which the poet's warm, tender, and touching concern had sought to keep me."

I embraced as a model for *Letters to a Young Iowan* the thoroughly democratic notion that in a country as small as Rilke's Germany, or a state as small as our own Iowa, a young citizen might dare to write the land's most famous son, and an abiding friendship might ensue. By the time I was through marking all the quotable passages in my book of Rilke—in the *library's* book—it looked like a Christmas tree generously decorated. Each lime green tab marked a spot in Rilke's letters where a passage of beauty or sorrow, wisdom or insight, bloomed. In the passion of the Rilke-Cappus exchange, roles of correspondent and correspondee became muddied: pupil become teacher, master turned apprentice. In the eighth letter, Rilke cautioned his young friend, "Do not believe that he who seeks to comfort you lives untroubled among the simple and quiet words that sometimes do you good."

The letter writers assembling to plumb the impenetrable depths of a young Iowan's psyche felt a similar trepidation. They wondered if they had earned the right to advise. They wondered if the gray hairs on their heads would render their message obsolete or otherwise unheard. Again, I thought of William Butler Yeats, a man as devoted to the small, green country of Ireland as we Iowans are to our small, green state, a man who had lamented his age in the poem "Among Schoolchildren," seeing himself as a mere "sixty-year-old smiling public man" among so many young and vibrant hearts. And though he fought his advancing years tooth and nail, Yeats knew the value of age. In "Sailing to Byzantium," he wrote,

> An aged man is but a paltry thing,
> A tattered coat upon a stick, unless
> Soul clap its hands and sing, and louder sing
> For every tatter in its mortal dress,
> Nor is there singing school but studying
> Monuments of its own magnificence.

Letters to a Young Iowan could do worse, I reckoned, than be a "singing school" for the monuments of Iowa's magnificence. Once welcomed, advice from older Iowans wary of living in glass houses flowed easily and freely. In lighter moments, I imagined the lot of us as the band the Village People doing a reunion tour, rocking it old-school: *Young Iowan, there's no need to feel down …*

Iowa makes dime-store philosophers of us all, it's true, a result, perhaps, of those long hours in the cornfields or schoolhouses … desk after desk, row upon row, mile after country mile pushing the brain to deeper thought. We are a state given to circumspection and best practice, to teaching and farming. We are devotees of the "right way," of "showing our math." We hold sacred those things we know could never be learned from a book—those swords and secrets we have swallowed, confessions and confidences made, wisdoms and wonders portrayed. Some day, we vow, when the time is right, we'll share those kernels of truth with some young soul sure to see them grow in the next generation. And, too often, we're not around to see the harvest.

By June, when the Chicago Cubs began their usual swoon, I had become aware that something special was in the works, and that this "little book" of letters had grown beyond me. I am always the last to know. I thought of Herman's Hermits crooning *Something tells me I'm into something good.* I found myself crossing the street whenever I espied one of the many black cats that mouse my Iowa town's crumbling grain elevators and abandoned buildings. *Get back, ye devils, get back.*

I had cat-scratch, letter-writing fever. In my mind I wrote and rewrote dozens of letters to young Iowans. It didn't matter whether I was bicycling or dishwashing or mowing. *Dear Young Iowan …* my thoughts began, the way a new camera makes its owner trigger-happy, the way a game of I-spy makes you see everything a certain color. I found myself paying close attention to the world around me, to its fine details, to its transience. Like Rilke's pal Franz Cappus, I had a hunch that letters beget poetry, and that the letters I was daily receiving from all corners of the state were working their own peculiar magic on their authors, and on me. I thought of former poet laureate Robert Pinsky's words in his essay "Poetry and Pleasure": "I have found it impossible to write a good personal letter without going at

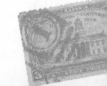

least a little further into myself than I might in conversation; the element of planning or composition seems to strip away barriers, props, and disguises, rather than to create them. I think we all find this true in letters from friends—even the brief hurried note seems to have concentrated some distillate of a person's inner nature."

In July, the book you now hold in your hands began to assume its final shape and garner some advance notice, as Mary Swander's letter appeared to rave reviews in the *Des Moines Register*. At last, I had all the pieces of the puzzle laid out before me, though I had yet to put them together. When I did, themes emerged. Patterns persisted. Concern for the environment, for diversity, for the farm—those quintessentially Iowan cares, came to the fore closely followed by education. Iowa oddities I particularly cheerleaded—letters that purported to reveal, for instance, what Iowa pigs have in common with Iowa men, how to translate the indecipherable language of spitting, why James T. Kirk hailed from Iowa, what love had to do, had to do with it.

How wide, I wondered, should the audience be? Should the book be titled simply *Letters to a Young Iowan* or should it reach out further to displaced Iowans and wanna-bes? After all, Iowa, for better and for worse, has always been known as a net exporter of people, good people. Historian Jon Gjerdge, a native Iowan now teaching at the University of California, Berkeley, tells us in his essay "Middleness and the Middle West" that in 1970, nearly 37 percent of Iowa-born Americans were living outside Iowa's borders. So many moved to California, in fact, that Southern Cal became known as the "Sea Coast of Iowa." Surely, a subtitle for *Letters to a Young Iowan* must acknowledge our brothers and sisters in exile. I flirted with *Letters to a Young Iowan: Advice from the Good Folks Who Brought You Grant Wood, Donna Reed, and Greg Brown*, but feared I might hear from angry heirs or product licensors. I weighed *Letters to a Young Iowan: How to Raise an Iowan Wherever You Are*, but thought it sounded too prescriptive, too Dr. Phil or Spock. Finally, I considered as a subtitle: *Epistles for Native Iowans and Those Who Want to Be*, but that seemed a bit too presumptuous. When combined with *Letters to a Young Iowan*, the subtitle *Good Sense from the Good Folks of Iowa for Young People Everywhere* seemed appropriately inclusive and inviting, two important Iowa virtues.

Who counts as an Iowan? This puzzler vexed from the beginning. How long does it take to speak Iowan, to feel Iowan, to be Iowan? Five years? Ten? Twenty-five? My call for "seasoned Iowans" brought on a number of confessions ... *Well, I was born in Missouri*, a contributor might say, *but I've lived here my whole adult life*, while another, raised in Iowa, had spent her adult life in another state and had returned as a retiree to drink deeply from the Iowa well. Like any good priest, I learned it was better to keep my mouth shut and the confessional open. Once rid of membership anxieties, most of the writers settled down to draft some mighty fine work. I figured the brand of contributor sufficiently thoughtful to query regarding their "Iowanness," and sufficiently rigorous in their introspection to question their geo-spiritual resumé, was a contributor I ought to hang onto in any case. Certainly, contributors had to make a permanent home in Iowa, at least part of the year—which left the door open for the growing number of retirees and semi-retirees who live in Iowa part-time (incidentally, one of many trends *Letters* uncovers). In a couple of cases, writers living in contiguous states were "in" by virtue of being honorary Iowans, someone we're proud to claim as our own, someone within shouting distance who returns when we call—someone like Iowa native Ted Kooser, who lives in Nebraska, or Jim Heynen, who lives in St. Paul. The goofiness of the membership question made me wonder, at times, whether inclusion might as well be based on some secret handshake, password, or trivia question: *What was the subject of Doctor Tom Davis' PhD dissertation? What's the lowest nine-hole score recorded by Iowa's weatherman-golfer extraordinaire, Denny Frary? Who was Iowa's first territorial governor? In 500 words or less, explicate the plot of the Iowa feature film* Zadar Cow from Hell.

Fortunately for me, the tone of the letters, thoroughly Iowan, resolved any lingering doubts: earnestness and gratefulness emerged predominant. But other feelings, too, were aired—fear for our privacies in an electronic age, anger at corporations, hurt over the War on Terror, righteousness in taking a spiritual stand, pride in preserving the family farm, honor for serving one's country in war, disgust at the excesses of the Boomer generation. But the most common feeling of all was hope—hope for what might be achieved when the old join forces with the young—and optimism for an unprecedented time in history when four generations of Iowans breathe

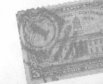

the same heady air. To that end, letter writers who grew up waltzing to the music of Iowa's Glenn Miller share these pages with those who grew up grooving to Iowa's Bo Ramsey and Greg Brown. There are familial legacies at work here, too: Greg Brown's daughter, Pieta, writing to the next generation of Iowa poets and songsmiths, for example; Myrna Sandvik and Ron Sandvik, mother and son, writing Iowa letters that appear side by side; couples Bruce and Jeanette Hopkins and Sharon and Tom Savage co-writing letters in the spirit of Sonny and Cher.

The various and sundry jobs of the contributors represent Iowa's occupational resourcefulness: journalists, musicians, politicians, extension agents, factory technicians, artists, professional athletes, historians, writers, friars, lawyers, nuns, museum directors, small business owners, farmers, engineers, speechwriters, park rangers, radio and television personalities, teachers, government employees. A quick glance through the table of contents reveals a former Governor, an Olympic champion, a nationally syndicated radio dramatist, a former U.S. Congressman, a former All-American, a former First Lady, an ex-Lieutenant Governor, a Grammy nominee, award-winning authors too numerous to mention, and, if the above fails to impress, a two-time winner of the Star Trek costume contest! To these folks, I am especially grateful, as lord knows fame makes the meditation requisite for a thoughtful letter especially difficult. From them, I have learned to be glad for my anonymity.

The subject matter of the letters is quite literally, and quite appropriately, *all over the map*. It reflects the mix Robert Pinsky talks up as the unique gift of letters—a combination of "news, musing, inquiry"—all perfectly pureed. Made from the flotsam and jetsam of a life richly lived in Iowa, letters like these are more well-built birds' nests than pre-fab condos, more twine and twig and mother's hair than rebar and composite board. In these letters, Iowans articulate Iowa's understated diversity—its overlooked African American history, its influential Native American folkways, its unconditional support for the gifted and the disabled, and its big-hearted embrace of religious and cultural difference. And in these letters Iowans remind us of our firm grasp of the fundamentals: food, farms, friends … love, learning, land, and longevity.

As I put the finishing touches on this introduction, *Letters* enters yet another season. Football is now upon us, along with two-a-day practices, referee shortages, and football media days. Summer shows signs of relenting. Some days it flares up red and angry; other days it merely huffs and puffs.

Such in-between times make good times for thinking, for letter writing—now when the seasons hang in the balance. I've always fancied the Roman god Janus, who had two faces looking in opposite directions—picture the masks of comedy and tragedy put back to back. Janus served as the god of gates and doors and of entrances and exits: one face looked into the past and the other looked into the future.

To be entering middle age as an Iowa farmer's son, as I am, means you see half of your life behind you—the good old days—and half in front—still better days to come … more strawberry malts in the summer, you resolve, more ice-skating and snowball fights in the winter. I have lived now in four of Iowa's counties. I grew up in Iowa's countryside and went on to live in its cities and small towns. I have gone to college here and elsewhere—enough, I think, to know what I don't know and be grateful for the mysteries that remain. I have put it in all in a letter, a letter sufficiently diverse in its wisdoms that I could not have hoped to write it all by myself.

If, God help us, *Letters to a Young Iowan* ever begets a monstrous sequel, something like *Godzilla*, I have taken the liberty of bequeathing some potential sequel subtitles. As with any Iowan, I rest assured only when my affairs are in order, when my wishes are known. To that end, I must say I quite like *Letters to a Young Iowan: Hayden Fry Returns*, though *Letters to a Young Iowan: Attack of the Killer Pork Chops* may better draw the teen crowd. Still, something a bit more *CSI*-snappy may be required, something like *LYI: The Iowa Hooverball Confederacy* or *LYI: The Bride of Frankenfood*.

Anyone for *Switchgrass Strikes Back?* Or, perhaps my favorite, *Letters to a Young Iowan: Children of the Corn(y)*.

Never say never.

Something serious remains to be said about the special pitfalls of a book like *Letters to a Young Iowan*, where the old presume to advise the young, and still more remains to be said about the virtues of such a risky and

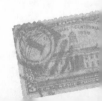

worthwhile proposition. I leave it to a better writer than I—Sherwood Anderson and his midwestern classic *Winesburg, Ohio*:

> The old man had listed hundreds of the truths in his book. I will not try to tell you of all of them. There was the truth of virginity and the truth of passion, the truth of wealth and of poverty, of thrift and of profligacy, of carelessness and abandon. Hundreds and hundreds were the truths and they were all beautiful ...
>
> It was the truths that made the people grotesques. The old man had quite an elaborate theory concerning the matter. It was his notion that the moment one of the people took one of the truths to himself, called it his truth, and tried to live his life by it, he became a grotesque and the truth he embraced became a falsehood.
>
> You can see for yourself how the old man, who had spent all of his life writing and was filled with words, would write hundreds of pages concerning this matter. The subject would become so big in his mind that he himself would be in danger of becoming a grotesque. He didn't ... It was the young thing inside him that saved the old man.

Letters to a Young Iowan, Part One
Last Names A-J

<table>
<tr><td>Jonathan G. Andelson</td><td>Lori Erickson</td></tr>
<tr><td>Duane Acker</td><td>Bob Everhart</td></tr>
<tr><td>Jim Autry</td><td>Timothy Fay</td></tr>
<tr><td>Marvin Bell</td><td>Hugh Ferrer</td></tr>
<tr><td>Pat Blank</td><td>Mary Flagel</td></tr>
<tr><td>Stephen G. Bloom</td><td>Susan Futrell</td></tr>
<tr><td>David Bock</td><td>Dan Gable</td></tr>
<tr><td>Dean Borg</td><td>Lois Swartzendruber Gugel</td></tr>
<tr><td>Daniel Brawner</td><td>Cary J. Hahn</td></tr>
<tr><td>Pieta Brown</td><td>Morgan Halgren</td></tr>
<tr><td>Donna Buell</td><td>David Hamilton</td></tr>
<tr><td>Tim Carman</td><td>Neil E. Harl</td></tr>
<tr><td>Scott Cawelti</td><td>Phyllis Harris</td></tr>
<tr><td>Mike Chapman</td><td>Phil Hey</td></tr>
<tr><td>Hal S. Chase</td><td>Jim Heynen</td></tr>
<tr><td>Kris Clark</td><td>Vicky Hinsenbrock</td></tr>
<tr><td>Dan Coffey</td><td>Bruce and Jeanette Hopkins</td></tr>
<tr><td>Thomas Burnell Colbert</td><td>Brion Hurley</td></tr>
<tr><td>Shirley Damsgaard</td><td>Patrick Irelan</td></tr>
<tr><td>Les Deal</td><td>Jan Jensen</td></tr>
<tr><td>Thomas K. Dean</td><td>Craig Johnson</td></tr>
<tr><td>Mark Edwards</td><td></td></tr>
</table>

Good Sense from the Good Folks of Iowa

Jonathan G. Andelson

Jonathan G. Andelson teaches anthropology and directs the Center for Prairie Studies at Grinnell College in Grinnell, Iowa, where he joined the faculty in 1974. Andelson was born in Chicago and grew up in nearby Evanston, Illinois. He earned his Bachelor's degree from Grinnell in 1970 and his Master's and Doctorate from the University of Michigan.

Dear Young Iowan:

Don't be afraid to get mud on your boots. Or what I really want to say is: get some mud on your boots. If the most fertile soil makes the best mud, then Iowa has some of the finest mud anywhere. That soil took thousands of years to make. Every year the prairie grew in the spring and summer and into the fall, then in winter died back to the roots. The litter decayed and sometimes burned, and the richness was returned to the soil. Every year, for thousands of years. For most of that time there were people here, helping the process. Then, three lifetimes ago, other people came, saw that the land was good, and began making new lives for themselves on it. Sadly, they took out most of the prairie to do it, and we've lost a lot of that rich soil. But you can still get some excellent mud on your boots, and that's a good start in connecting yourself to the land.

There are a lot of ways to do it. Come with me and do a little rambling through the remaining bits of prairie. (Do you know how to ramble? A lot of people these days don't seem to know how, but it isn't hard. Just look down and put one foot in front of the other.) In the prairie different flowers bloom every week during the summer and early fall, and some of the prairie grasses are six or seven feet high. We might see butterflies, beetles, bluebirds, grouse, prairie crayfish, even a coyote or fox if we're lucky. I keep hoping to see a prairie chicken. With some friends and neighbors I am also helping to restore some prairie, to bring a little wildness back to Iowa.

But find your own favorite way to connect with the land. Maybe it's making a garden grow, or crops, or turkey hunting, or hunting for mushrooms in the fall, or closely observing wildlife, or picking wild berries, or caring for

Good Sense from the Good Folks of Iowa

horses or other outdoor animals, or hiking or biking or camping. You can connect with the land deeply by going caving. You can connect with the land on the water, too. Try fishing, or canoeing, or kayaking, or sailboating. (There, I've shown you my bias. I think you can connect with the land better when you aren't using a motor.) You can also connect with the land in the winter. Snow on your boots counts just as well as mud in my challenge to you. Make a snow angel or an igloo. Try skiing, especially the cross-country kind.

Connect with the land through *all* of your senses. Taste the tingly leaf of the mountain mint that grows on the prairie; it makes a good tea. Relish the vegetables fresh from a garden. Listen to the crickets at night and reckon the temperature (count the chirps in 14 seconds and add 40). Listen to the snow. (When I walk on hard snow on a cold day it sounds to me like *kyurng-kyurng-kyurng*. What snow sounds can you hear?) Get down on your knees and smell the soil, especially after a rain, and of course take time to smell the flowers—though not all of them smell. Touch the soil. Is it crumbly loam, hard and chunky clay, or silky silt? Touch feathery moss, the smooth leaves of a corn plant (warning: sharp edges), and the sandpapery leaves of a compass plant or a cup plant on the prairie. Don't touch poison ivy. And of course use your eyes to see the land's beauty: everything from the microscopic beauty of a dragonfly wing, to a geode, to an oat field, to the vast beauty of the night sky.

Life goes on without television, or computer games, or iPods. The thing is, life does not go on without the land. But for the land to go on we must take care of it, and to take care of it we must both know it and value it. Connecting to the land is the beginning of knowing and valuing it. So get out in the land, really *in* it. Get your boots (or your shoes or your bare feet) muddy—or dusty, or snowy, or wet. But please wipe your boots off before you come back in and tell me about it.

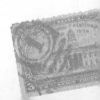

Duane Acker

Dr. Duane Acker returned to operate his family farm near Atlantic, Iowa, in 1993 after serving as administrator of the Foreign Agricultural Service and assistant secretary for science and education in the U.S. Department of Agriculture (USDA) in Washington, D.C. Since then he has lectured widely and reviewed agricultural programs in several states as well as China, Costa Rica, Belarus, Ukraine, and the Republic of Georgia.

Dr. Acker's major career was in universities. He taught animal science at Oklahoma State University and Iowa State University, was associate dean of agriculture at Kansas State University, dean at South Dakota State University, vice chancellor at the University of Nebraska and, for eleven years, president of Kansas State University. He has authored two books, Animal Science and Industry *and* Can State Universities Be Managed?

Dear Young Iowan:

This past March, the thirty-year-old manager of a Florida residential community where we winter came to me with a litany of frustrations—city and county regulations, indecisive staff in the corporation that developed the community, incomplete project cost estimates, misunderstandings with contractors, late material deliveries, and work not completed on time. Most community board meetings had become gripe sessions about unfinished projects.

He asked how I'd managed to complete the projects I'd taken on as a member of the board.

Years earlier I'd been asked the same question after leading a USDA agency out of severe budget problems. We had combined multiple units, cancelled auto and equipment leases, and out-placed surplus staff to other agencies.

I'd been asked the same question in universities, after we'd closed some long-time research projects and instituted an English language screening process for graduate teaching assistants. *How did you get things changed that tradition had kept in place?*

I grew up on a small Iowa farm where animals had to be fed, cows milked, and eggs gathered twice a day. Every machine and person had its limit. I just learned that one has to get things done within whatever limits exist. This is what I said in response to that Florida community manager.

On the Iowa farm of my youth, corn had to be planted by early May, and alfalfa had to be harvested in the early bud stage for best feeding value. We had to get maximum production and income from every acre and every animal.

We had financial limits, as we had mostly borrowed our operating funds. Every machine the farm business could afford—tractor, grinder, mower, milking machine, baler—had its constraints. Every crop and every animal had its genetic limit. Rainfall and soil fertility also constrained. My father, our hired worker, and I each had physical and time limits. Except for Saturday and Sunday and the summer months, my work had to be done before I got on the school bus at 7:45 and after I got home at 4:30.

My response to our community manager was that he simply needed to decide which "regulations" applied, talk directly to decision-makers and doers, double-check project specifications and target dates, sometimes find a substitute tool or material that would work, make decisions others would not make, and, if a key worker didn't show, grab a spade, a hammer, or a telephone and do the job himself.

Much of management—of a business, an organization, a project, or even of oneself—is reducing real constraints and ignoring imagined ones. With equipment, we read the instruction manual, lubricate, adjust, and maintain all parts in good condition. With animals, we feed and care for comfort and production. With crops, we prepare a good seedbed, fertilize, and protect from pests. Over the long term, in the case of both crops and animals, we make genetic improvement.

With people, we train well and compassionately. We reduce administrative layers and eliminate redundant paperwork, meetings, or clearances. We make decisions in areas of responsibility, and we reward initiative and good work completed on time.

The starting point for achieving an organization's full potential is the individual who clearly sees the organization's purpose, capacities, and

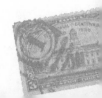

constraints, then makes the needed decisions and takes the necessary actions.

For these things to happen, the person—likely you, young Iowan—must first believe that you can do anything you really want to do. Second, develop those critical skills—physical, mental, communication, and personal relationship skills—and especially self-confidence. Third, learn from, but be unfettered by, tradition. Fourth, do what you can do best, and let others do what they can do better. Fifth, celebrate when you win; learn when you lose.

That Iowa farm of my youth and other early experiences, including day work on neighbors' farms and driving the school bus my senior year, each gave me the responsibility to get things done well, on time, and within existing constraints. Experiences later in life—in universities, government agencies, businesses, and, eventually, back to operate that Iowa farm (by then more than one thousand acres and marketing corn, soybeans, alfalfa, and beef)—gave plenty of evidence that I should be thankful for that early Iowa farm experience, especially the patience, guidance, and confidence of my parents and others of that rural community.

If you grow up in an environment comparable in work experience, guidance, and confidence-building, whether on an Iowa farm or in a village or city, you are fortunate. See that you make the most of it!

Sincerely yours,

Duane Acker

Jim Autry

Jim Autry is the retired president of the Meredith Magazine Group, where he enjoyed a distinguished career as an editor and publisher. Autry has been active in many civic, charitable, and arts organizations over a thirty-year period, including serving as president, chairman, and chairman emeritus of the Epilepsy Foundation of America, a founding member of the board of People for the American Way, and the co-founder of the Des Moines National Poetry Festival. Autry is the author of eight books, with a ninth and tenth forthcoming, as well as a frequent contributor to magazines and anthologies nationwide. He was a featured poet in Bill Moyers' 1989 PBS series, The Power of the Word, *and Garrison Keillor has featured his work on* The Writer's Almanac.

Autry received his BA in Journalism from the University of Mississippi and has since been awarded three honorary degrees. In 1997-98, he held an endowed chair in leadership at Iowa State University, and he continues to consult and speak on leadership in America and abroad, efforts which have earned him the Lifetime Service to the Public Humanities award from the Iowa Humanities Board. He says that his real claim to fame is that he is married to Iowa's former Lieutenant Governor, Sally Pederson.

Dear Young Iowan:

At age twenty-two and now graduating from a special college program, you have already benefited greatly from the community we call "Iowa." Although we don't talk about this with you, and you are only casually aware of it, you have had autism since you were an infant, and you will have it all your life.

"Having autism" means different things to different people, depending on their cluster of symptoms, but this letter is not about autism itself; it's about what it means to have autism, or any other disability, in Iowa. Thus, this letter is about Iowa, because had you been born in my home state of Mississippi—or in any of another dozen states I could name—you likely would not be graduating from a college program. You might even be living in an institution.

But Iowa has given you an advantage in this world; Iowa has given you the benefits of a splendid public education, an education available to all

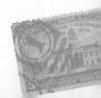

students whether rich or poor, black or white or yellow or brown, able or disabled.

When you were two-and-a-half years old, the Des Moines public schools sent an "infant intervention" teacher to our home to help you learn to play and develop motor skills. You started preschool before you were three years old. You have participated fully in school: playing in the band, running track, and enjoying social events. You were not the best musician and you were not the fastest runner, but you were part of the ensemble and you were in the race.

I'm happy you want to make your home in Iowa, and I hope and pray that you will realize your dream of finding a life partner and having children. This won't be easy for you, as it is not easy for anyone with a disability, but if it's possible anyplace, it's possible in Iowa.

Despite our state's continuing problems and the need to always be improving, Iowa still offers the most supportive environment I can imagine for living, working, and raising a family. And Iowans themselves have a positive attitude about these things. They will want you to accomplish your goals and will do what they can to help you personally. Of course, you've already experienced this generous spirit and you know there is every reason for you to continue to experience it.

But what you have to do in return is to continue to be the generous and loving person that you are, helping and supporting others. That's the bargain we make as Iowans: everyone has the responsibility to the best of his or her ability to contribute to this great community, to be willing to help others, and to be an active part of accomplishing our shared goals. Every Iowan, even those with disabilities, must be committed to a better life here for everyone, not just for themselves. That's the deal.

I know I can count on you, Ronald. And you can count on Iowa.

Love,

Dad

Marvin Bell

Marvin Bell served two terms as Iowa's first Poet Laureate. He has published nineteen books of poetry and essays, the latest being Mars Being Red *in 2007. Mr. Bell taught forty years for the Iowa Writers' Workshop, retiring in 2005 as Flannery O'Connor Professor of Letters. In 2006, he was named a Distinguished Alumnus of the University of Iowa. He now teaches for the low-residency MFA program based at Pacific University in Oregon. He and his wife, Dorothy, split the year between Iowa City and Port Townsend, Washington. He has a son in New York City and a son and grandchildren in Signal Mountain, Tennessee.*

Dear Young Iowan:

Aren't you tired of being given advice? I'd be. I was. Grown-ups have a habit of telling others how to live. Let's be candid. One decides how to act by watching how others act, and the consequences, not by listening to what they say. I'll limit myself to one suggestion so, when you come up with the same idea, you'll know someone else also thinks it a good one. Here it comes.

Go somewhere.

Now, I may get a nasty letter from the same Iowa governmental office that went begging former Iowans living in California to please come home, but I am of the mind that a young person ought to follow the motto of the mongoose in Rudyard Kipling's "Rikki-Tikki-Tavi": "Run and find out." This country is bigger and more diverse than you can imagine. Many, many people believe that they live in the best place. Well, our judgments of a place are in part our judgments of ourselves. And wherever you go, you take yourself along. So take yourself somewhere.

And when you get there, you will be asked to explain Iowa. Or tempted to, each time someone meeting you for the first time says, "Oh, I have a friend in Columbus," or "I love your potatoes." Face it, perhaps because America is vast and powerful, Americans are provincial, and those who live on the coasts are doomed never to know the richness of this country. Go somewhere. Go many somewheres. If and when you return, you will be a

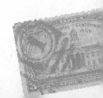

bigger person inside. You will carry a thousand secret smiles. You will not feel you missed the boat.

I myself am not keen to explain Iowa to my coastal pals. After all, where would one stop? You'd have to explain that Iowa is not Indiana, and Kansas is not Ohio, Colorado is not near New Mexico, and Illinois is more than Chicago. I generally content myself with pointing out that one needs gears on one's bicycle in most of Iowa, that it is beautiful in four seasons, that it is neither as cold in winter as the North nor as hot in summer as the South, that Iowans generally believe in education, and that we are largely independent political thinkers. Hence, we have often had, among our Congressmen and Senators, both a conservative and a liberal, and sometimes on the electoral map, Iowa will be a blue interruption.

Iowa is a great state for farmers, for country mice, for the civic-minded and the tolerant, for those who believe in the value of education, and for those who can't be pigeon-holed. It's also a good place for writers. Iowa has tons of corn and soybeans and acres of writers.

Why is Iowa a good place for writers? Well, partly because of what it is and where, but also because of what it is not and where it is not. Literary careers are made and unmade in major cities on the coasts. But literature— the actual writing—is made all over the country. It can be difficult to see one's art clearly in the midst of the hubbub of literary careerism.

I don't know what it means to come from Iowa. I come from a village on the south shore of eastern Long Island. But I know what it means to like Iowa and to stay here.

Maybe you want to stay put. That's fine, too. If you read books. One always lives locally, but one's consciousness can range from coast to coast, and cross the oceans, and ring the globe. Remember Mark Twain's remark that the man (or woman) who does not read has no advantage over the man (or woman) who cannot read. Nothing will so much affect your life as your ability with language. It gets you a job and a raise, a date and a spouse, the best friends, and practical advantages too numerous to list.

I'm not going to tell you that you have to stay in Iowa. Iowa deserves to prosper, but attracting and retaining residents is not your assignment. Your assignment is to increase your options, to find out what you didn't know

11

you knew, to live fully, to pay attention to your inner life, and to do good works as much as possible.

So. Go somewhere. And be *from* somewhere.

Your fan, Marvin Bell (The Geezer)

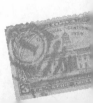

Pat Blank

Pat Blank is a senior news producer for Iowa Public Radio's KUNI. She grew up on a farm in north central Iowa with her parents and two brothers, and later attended Iowa Lakes Community College in Estherville and the University of Northern Iowa in Cedar Falls. She lives on an acreage just outside Shell Rock with her husband, yellow Lab, five cats and sixteen pygmy goats.

Dear Young Iowan:

Sometimes it's important to take stock, to count your blessings or count your chickens, though, of course, not before they hatch.

Having lived in Iowa all my life, I think back to my childhood years from time to time and those thoughts bring a smile to my face. I remember how alfalfa smells just after it's baled and how we worked from sunrise to sunset to get it in the barn before the rain came. Several neighbors came to help, and, when the crop filled the barn to bulging, we left the top door open just a crack to let it "breathe," much the same way you loosen your belt after a Thanksgiving feast. We celebrated our haymaking with a late supper, including lemonade made with real lemons and sugar.

In the middle of summer, small-town celebrations like "Sauerkraut Days," "Sweetcorn Days," and "Beef Days" provided a bit of respite from all the farm chores. They offered a chance to see friends, family, and neighbors—those people who are sometimes overly curious about your life but who are always the first to organize a soup supper or benefit auction if someone is sick and needs money for medical bills. These are the same folks who, in the fall, will harvest the crops of an injured farmer or recent widow before they do their own.

Eating establishments in little towns were and still are often family-owned with a lunch special everyday featuring mashed potatoes, some type of meat, and pie for dessert. Coffee there is just plain coffee—no special flavorings or foam—and it's less than a dollar a cup with free refills. Just help yourself.

Good Sense from the Good Folks of Iowa

If the cafe is closed or too full and it's raining, look for the farmers at the co-op elevator. They'll be drinking coffee and playing a dice game with die shaken from a plastic cup. In the fall they'll be discussing how much moisture the corn has or how good the soybean yield is.

So, if you decide to leave Iowa for a couple of years, know that you'll be welcomed back at any time with open arms and familiar sights. You'll know when you cross the state line because everyone waves.

And when summer finally rolls around again, young Iowan, pull off the beaten path, turn off the radio, and roll down the windows. If you listen closely, you might just hear the corn grow.

Sincerely,

Pat Blank

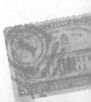

Stephen G. Bloom

Since 1993, Stephen Bloom has taught at the University of Iowa, where he specializes in narrative journalism. Bloom is co-founder of The Oxford Project *with photographer Peter Feldstein, examining life in the rural community of Oxford, Iowa. Bloom's most decorated book,* Postville: A Clash of Cultures in Heartland America, *also intimately concerns an Iowa community.* Postville *was named a Best Book of the Year by MSNBC,* Chicago Sun-Times, Denver Rocky Mountain News, Chicago Tribune, *and* St. Louis Post-Dispatch.

Bloom has worked as a staff writer for the Los Angeles Times, Dallas Morning News, Sacramento Bee *and* San Jose Mercury News. *His freelance stories have appeared in* Smithsonian, DoubleTake, Points of Entry, The Washington Post, Chicago Tribune Magazine, *and* New York Times Magazine. *He currently is under contract with St. Martin's Press to write* Tears of Mermaids: The Secret History of Pearls, *a nonfiction detective story.*

Dear Young Iowan:

Here are "Twenty-five Things All Young Iowans Need To Know."

1. As soon as you can, travel. Travel out of state. Travel to New York and California. Travel to Europe, Asia and South America. Iowa is a homogenous state. However good Iowa schools are, you will learn more by meeting people who are different from you—different looking and different thinking.

2. Despite what your parents and grandparents probably taught you—that children should be seen and not heard—that only goes so far. To succeed in the larger world, you can't be shy or quiet. Fiercely advocate for yourself and your abilities.

3. Read. *The Travels of Marco Polo* is a good start. So is *On the Road*. At the least, go to Iowa City for a reading at Prairie Lights Books.

4. While there, stop in at Atlas, 126, or Hamburg Inn, all within a few blocks.

Good Sense from the Good Folks of Iowa

Pretend you're sipping on a *citron presse* at La Coupole or Le Dome, two famous writers' haunts in Paris.

5. Try not to work at the local grocery store. As a teenager, you'll probably think the money is good, but you can do more with your time than sacking groceries.

6. Work hard in high school to master Spanish. Spanish will be essential to your success whether you stay in Iowa or move elsewhere. Take advantage of any field trips or exchange programs to foreign countries your high school offers.

7. Write for your high school newspaper. If the clique of kids at the paper bugs you, start your own.

8. Learn how to play a musical instrument. Before you choose which one, make sure you like how it sounds and how it feels in your hands.

9. Realize there will always be people cooler than you.

10. Take chances. Chat up the girl or boy you have a crush on. The worst that can happen is you'll get ignored, and you'll realize the object of your affection wasn't worth your attention.

11. "Do what you love and the money will follow" isn't bad advice.

12. At garage sales outside of Iowa, you are expected to bargain.

13. Kids who are dopers are losers. Drinking is not cool. Don't drive with someone who does either. Chances are not slim that you will get into an accident, maybe a fatal one.

14. Get yourself to Des Moines to visit the two best museums in Iowa—the State Historical Museum and the Des Moines Art Center.

15. If you can convince your parents to go, the Art Institute and the Field Museum in Chicago are terrific places in which to get lost. While in Chicago, eat deep-dish pizza. Make sure you go on St. Patrick's Day to see the Chicago River dyed green.

16. Write a short story about someone who cracks you up.

17. Life is a series of distinct moments. Be aware when they happen.

18. Remember that not everyone is Christian.

19. If you move to a large city, learn some Yiddish. *Chutzpah, shtik, moxie, macher, mishpokhe,* and *mensch* is a good beginning. If you want to learn more, get Leo Rosten's *Joys of Yiddish.*

20. Be aware that if you move from Iowa, people might not know that supper and dinner are different; that pop and soda are the same; what seven-layer salad, Maid-Rite sandwiches, and mudrooms are; and that you visit *with* someone. No one will know (or care) about the differences between coveralls and overalls. Carhartts are to Iowans what Ikea is to Californians.

21. Don't smoke. It's an expensive habit, will make you smell, and likely will shorten your life. It'll also burn holes in your shirts.

22. While in Iowa City, go to the University Art Museum and sit in front of the Jackson Pollock painting. Study it.

23. Autumn bonfires and hayrack rides are fun, but don't forget to bring a blanket.

24. Fully engage in whatever you do. Don't do anything half-throttle.

25. Outside of Iowa, there's no need to correct those who confuse Iowa with Ohio and Idaho. It's all the same to them.

David Bock

David Bock was born in 1939 in Chicago, where he completed his secondary and college education. After a year of graduate study in philosophy at the University of Toronto, he entered New Melleray Abbey, a Cistercian-Trappist monastery near Peosta, in 1962. Bock further studied theology at the monastery and later in Dubuque, Iowa, where he was ordained a priest in 1976 and served the Abbey as its superior and abbot until 1984. Father Bock is now the librarian and cook for the New Melleray community, as well as an occasional teacher in the Abbey. He serves as a member of the Board of Monastic Interreligious Dialogue, which promotes exchanges among monasteries of world religions.

Dear Young Iowan:

> *God Spoke to Job Out of a Storm*—Job 38:1

Our society expends a huge amount of effort and money to remove and recycle the mountains of garbage and waste that survive our consumer-oriented lifestyles. Outside of Iowa and too often within it, "waste" has a bad name. The very idea of waste seems destructive of our goals of productivity and efficiency. Wasted time and effort are a shame. Wasted lives and minds are tragedies.

It is hard to shift into modes of communication and activity that seem to *need* waste to function. We forgive nature its wastefulness: the prodigality and abundance of our fertile fields and woods, for example. We ignore its cycles of destructiveness and degeneration until sometimes we are struck by a devastating storm. The storm lays waste; it devastates. Our language links the unbounded sense contained in both *waste* and *vast*. Creative works of art and poetry mimic nature in asking us to dispense with our demands for productivity and efficiency.

We Iowans are trained to focus on the essential, to extract objective facts from what we observe. We are provided with "news capsules" and headings that tell us "all we need to know." Art and poetry, it seems, just take too much time. We don't just stand before them as detached observers who ask questions of them or make judgments; poetry and works of art ask questions of us. They ask us to hear the questions and hear the emotions they probe. We are invited to enter into a sphere of stillness and silence so that we can hear the words as they are uttered and so that we can hear our own response. Silence may be less frightening to stoic Iowans who—perhaps—better know the vastness of unsuspected depths borne in hearts. Still, we usually prefer to shield ourselves from this unknown side of ourselves. But sometimes it emerges with the intensity of a storm rising from the sea.

Poetry can help us to communicate with our inner depths. It has a capacity to unveil what is usually hidden, even though it is lying right under our feet. In his book *A Timbered Choir: The Sabbath Poems, 1979-1997*, Wendell Berry seems to open our eyes to the rhythm and flow of nature which disappears even as it manifests itself. He writes of a pair of swallows who, "With tender exactitude / Play out their line / In arcs laid out on the air, / As soon as made, not there." Are the swallows wasteful in their flight? Or is theirs an abundance which cannot be possessed or held? Another poet, Marianne Moore, speaks in her poem "Keeping Their World Large" of "A noiseless piano, an innocent war, the heart that can act against itself." She overlays seemingly paradoxical images which plunge us into self-awareness: the potential lurking in us to yield to the deepest deceit and greatest waste of "the heart that can act against itself."

God often speaks as a poet, ready to engage our hearts. However, we are sometimes given "condensed" versions of the truth conveyed by God's words. It takes "too much time" to listen to these words as poetry, to be silent before them, and to let them rouse a spirit within us. There is "too much subjectivity," some say, in this approach.

But it seems worthwhile to let God be a poet, and not a mechanic or dogmatist. Is creation a mechanism or is it a poem? One has to be patient to read or write a poem. The process is a slow unfolding that involves waiting for different parts of reality to come to their own maturity. We recognize that we may read for a long time without understanding. If understanding does come, it may come only later. Poets often write a lifetime without being understood or appreciated. But the labor of poetry—reading or writing—is somehow its own justification. The labor of living is somehow its own justification. Productivity, results, acclaim from others are false criteria in this most crucial matter of living our own lives. We are called to act out of our own truth and the worst betrayal is "the heart that can act against itself."

Poetry dares to confront the deepest forces of destructiveness and evil. It sometimes makes us uncomfortable as it pulls down those screens that prevent our acknowledging reality's contingencies. Disruptive and destructive forces, we must recall, are as much a part of life as the constructive and comfortable. Religion incorporates the struggle with evil, sin, and illusion into its vision of reality. This conflict leads us into a wholeness that is mature enough to embrace all of our lives. We discover from within that we participate in a vast unfolding of life that exceeds our comprehension but which invites our commitment.

If God is a poet, we Iowans must yield to a slow, patient, laborious unfolding of a work in life which will reveal its full meaning only when it is complete. It is easier, but mistaken, to compromise—to think that what we do and say has no effect on our inner self. We know the capacity of our heart to act against itself. We also know the life-giving energy that comes from words and action uttered from the depths of personal being. When we speak and listen from these depths, we know we are in communion with the pervasive and embracing reality of God's work that is bringing about our own wholeness and the wholeness of the world.

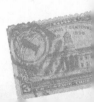

Dean Borg

Raised on a Winnebago County farm and educated in a one-room country school, Dean Borg has combined news and public affairs in a more than forty-year career as a broadcast journalist. His distinguished work as a producer for Iowa Public Television and Iowa Public Radio has earned him the coveted title senior correspondent.

Borg, who was voted "outstanding boy" by his graduating high school class in Forest City, holds degrees from the University of Iowa and Iowa State University, which has honored him as a distinguished alumni—the highest award given by the University to its alumni. Dean and his wife Sheila live in Mount Vernon with their daughter Kierstyn. The family also includes four sons, three of whom are Air Force officers and a fourth who has earned the title doctor of animal science.

Dear Young Iowan:

You'll hear all sorts of slogans promoting Iowa, including such well-meaning catchphrases as "Fields of Opportunity," "A Place to Grow," and "A State of Minds." Although "Iowa—You Make Me Smile" fell into disfavor, I wasn't among its detractors. I do feel a sort of smugness about living here.

I've been incredibly fortunate to have spent most of my life in Iowa, but I've also traveled throughout the world enough to be convinced how really lucky I am. On several occasions, my sons have commented how, when driving into Iowa after an extended time in distant states, they sense a difference in the ambiance and even the air they breathe as they moved northward along Interstate 35 from Iowa's southern border.

Because Iowa's rural and urban cultures are so closely integrated, I'm able to enjoy the best of both worlds. I prize my heritage of growing up on a farm—learning a work ethic that ignores the clock and defines the work day by essential tasks completed. I remember working well past sundown, picking up baled hay from a field that was illuminated only by flashes of lightning from an approaching storm—a storm we had to beat to save the day—and the hay.

Iowa gives me space. Anywhere in Iowa, whether in a corporate board room or broadcast studio, I'm only minutes away from green fields stretching to the horizon.

Good Sense from the Good Folks of Iowa

But I also have space to think, to plan, to dream. That may seem a contradiction to Iowans' work ethic, but in reality working and dreaming are complementary. While as a youth I worked what now seems incredibly hard on Iowa's farms and mowing Iowa's ditches, I was indeed getting a hands-on education in philosophy and life skills from men and women who were far from college professors.

Perhaps the most important character trait I learned as a young apprentice alongside laborers, and later professional mentors, is the absolute and unequivocal necessity for honesty and integrity. That character trait is the foundation of my career as a journalist because integrity nurtures trust. News sources must trust me with sensitive, often personal information. Those who hear my reports trust my ability to provide accurate and unbiased reporting. Working and socializing with men and women beyond the pressroom, studio, or classroom, have taught me to respect all people. In return, I have been trusted by people when reporting sometimes tense and desperate situations.

Trust has been shown me during interviews with victims of violent crime or weather tragedies, where raw nerves are exposed. That trust pays dividends during election season, when I am often honored to moderate high-stakes debates broadcast on television or radio. I particularly recall the televised, contentious debate between incumbent Iowa Senator John Culver and challenger Charles Grassley who was then a U.S. Representative. As the candidates sought political advantage—much like boxers in a title fight—viewers at home trusted me to enforce the rules equitably and to ask tough questions that cut through the rhetoric.

In the end, I think I know the real Iowa that transcends a tract on a map. Iowa is people—smart, caring, hard-working people who genuinely treasure and nurture each other. We find value in people, and we learn from them.

That's the heritage that energizes my life. Fortunately, it's still here for any young Iowan.

Sincerely,

Dean Borg

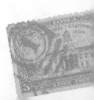

Daniel Brawner

Daniel Brawner was born and raised in rural Linn County and educated at Cornell College, Creighton University, and Arizona State University. He has been a freelance writer for many years, and for the past fifteen years he has served as an award-winning humor columnist for the Mount Vernon-Lisbon Sun. *Brawner is the author of the humorous mystery novel* Employment Is Murder *and is currently working on a spooky and spiritual musical, entitled* More, *about the excesses of consumerism.*

Dear Young Iowan:

Okay, I know I don't have the right to give you advice. I'm no shining example of success myself and I haven't exactly kept up with the latest details of your life—at least not as much as I would have wanted. And I know I'm not as smart as you are—but then, neither are most of the rest of the people on earth.

So here it is: go out and be the best you can be. You have my permission. Stop holding back. Let 'er rip! And don't tell me competitiveness is anti-social or unenlightened or any of the rest of that pacifist, New Age crap my sister drummed into your head during that brief period when you were still trainable. And don't tell me you've risen above unworthy pursuits like leaving your classmates speechless and choking on your dust as you set unreachable new records. Remember, I knew you before you knew yourself. You love that stuff!

I remember when you were just four years old and small for your age. We were having Thanksgiving with my uncle, that big Lakota Sioux who talked like Robert Mitchum. You and I were playing basketball in his driveway. Except you were too little to get the ball all the way to the hoop. But that didn't stop you from trying—over and over and over. Even when they called us for dinner, you refused to come in until you had made one basket. I watched you out of the window as you stood there, cold and hungry, summoning one hundred percent of your strength again and again, imagining you could command the ball to go through the hoop by force of will. You never did make a basket and you lost out on a good Thanksgiving dinner. But you won my respect that day.

Of course, your mom was always gushing about her boy genius. She bragged how you were doing trigonometry in fourth grade, or reading two thousand words a minute. I knew that was true because one time you came over to check out my new computer. You were barely big enough to see over the desk. I was trying to locate a particular file, but the new processor was so fast that when I brought up the directory, it went by in a blur. "It's there," you said quietly. I hadn't even been able to make out the words. But you had read and remembered the entire directory in a flash. I thought to myself, *This is no ordinary kid.*

I heard the stories about how you could throw a baseball so hard it would hurt the other kids' hands and they didn't want to play with you any more. But you refused to throw softer. So you quit Little League instead.

When you blazed through complicated math problems, your teacher in that silly, private high school you attended insisted you show how you arrived at the answers. You said you didn't know how and what difference did it make anyway? I've lost track of the number of times you dropped out of school or were kicked out for refusing to plod along with the other students.

Don't be afraid of your own power. Friedrich Nietzsche wrote, "Be careful, lest in casting out demons, you cast out the best thing that is in you." All right, so you're obstinate, imperious, resentful of authority, and you don't play well with others. So what? I'm sure they said the same about Alexander the Great. And if he'd been nothing but a sweet guy, his enemies would have left his bones to bleach on some battlefield long before he had conquered every nation in the known world.

As you consider your future, remember where you came from. You are the descendant of pioneers who left their sensible friends and comfortable homes in New England to scratch out a hard-scrabble living on the Iowa prairie. They were tough. They were stubborn. By the looks of those old tintype photos, some of them were even pretty mean. But they had to be to fight off the drought and the grasshoppers and the long hours of isolation. So if you find yourself restless and dissatisfied with the way things are, well, you come by it honestly.

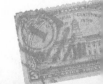

Your great-great-grandfather on my father's side left Ireland with its rotting potatoes and religious persecution to make his fortune in Iowa when all he had were the clothes on his back and the unrealistic conviction that he was going to get rich or whip any man who said it wasn't so.

Your great-great-grandfather Wesley on my mother's side fought in the Spanish-American War. It took him three weeks to reach the Philippines by ship. And as is characteristic of so many in our family, he was prone to motion sickness. The captain told him not to worry. After a couple of days, he'd get used to it. Wesley threw up everyday for three weeks until they came mercifully to port in Manila.

It wasn't long until one day they were out on patrol when a sniper, hiding in a tree shot Wesley's captain through the heart. He then proceeded to kill both of his friends, again, cleanly through the heart. That sniper was a terrific shot. But he wasn't perfect. He got your great-great-grandfather in the heart, too. But the bullet lodged in a bit of fat and failed to penetrate the organ itself.

Somehow Wesley's buddies got him back to camp and then onto the ship heading for home. The bullet was too close to the heart to operate, so the doctor just stuck him in a bathtub, packed with ice to keep him from bleeding to death. He regained consciousness and overheard the doctor tell the nurse, "Give him anything he wants to eat. He'll be dead by morning."

The doctor managed to save Wesley's life that night — and not because he was a terrific surgeon—but because he made your great-great-grandfather mad.

"I'll outlive that son of a bitch!" Wesley said to himself. And he did.

The Army doctors had told Wesley that bullet was still going to kill him some day. They warned his fiancée not to marry him. "One day, Wesley's heart is going to explode," they told her. "And you'll be a young widow." Fortunately for you and all of us, Madre was just as stubborn and true as Wesley. They ignored the well-intended advice and beat the odds by luck and hard work and uncompromising love. And, forty some years after they were married, that sniper's slow bullet finally reached Wesley's contented old heart. But it was too late to affect the outcome. Wesley had already won the game.

What I'm trying to tell you is that you might just as well give in to that fierce competitive impulse. It's in your blood. No matter how they might try back at the stables to harness him to the plow, a thoroughbred is born to run. So give it all you've got and don't worry about disappointing those who envision your future as accommodating and serene. You need to wake up that demon inside that made other kids afraid of you. Because he's your best friend. Your competitive demon is going to make you successful and respected. He might even make you rich. But mostly, he's going to make you happy.

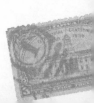

Pieta Brown

The daughter of two preachers' kids, Pieta Brown spent her childhood in a bohemian and musical family. During her early childhood in Iowa, Pieta was exposed to rural and traditional folk music, and country blues through her father, folk singer Greg Brown. Later, growing up in Alabama with a full-time working mother, Pieta expanded and drew on these influences, writing poetry and composing songs for piano.

Rambling in her early 20s, Pieta picked up a guitar and put her influences together in what quickly became the songs on her first, self-titled release in 2002. Now touring nationally, Brown often works with highly respected guitarist and producer, and fellow Iowan, Bo Ramsey. Her own mixture of country, rock, folk, and blues has prompted numerous comparisons to predecessors Bob Dylan, Rickie Lee Jones, Bobbie Gentry, the Carter Family, Lucinda Williams, and Tom Waits.

Dear Young Iowan:

I woke this morning from a dream of you standing in the field by the house where I lived when I was a young girl. You were standing there looking up at me as I read you a letter about days gone by: *The house where we lived was red. In summer it was covered in morning glories and the dogs ran free. There was a rusty pump in the front yard where we drew water for drinking and cooking and baths in a small metal tub. We had an outhouse and a run-down porch. It was a long ways to the nearest town. The streets were just gravel roads—and corn rows...* In the dream the letter was long, but you stood there to listen, knowing I was trying to get at something.

These days, even wide awake, I still find myself walking the streets of my teenage years. After moving all over the country, the different strains of my family moved back to Iowa, into town, to streets lined with old houses, and cars and small gardens in the summertime. After leaving home at eighteen, I moved all over the country again and then, as if I had already known before leaving, back to Iowa to a busy street lined with modest houses, and cars and small gardens in the summertime.

Now, every so often I drive outside of town to walk down the avenues of music, along small fields of lullabies where no translation is needed. No radio here. No television.

In the song there is the field, and the small towns falling apart or getting bigger with gray and tan developments, and dusty back roads, and the sun going up and coming down, and all the people working hard at all the things they do. There is a familiar, plaintive melody as old as the ground, falling like rain to run through the dirt back out to the rivers and streams that give borders to our lives.

It is here, along one of these borders, looking out across a field, I see new and worn machines and ghosts of mules and trees that look like hands. I see black clouds of birds on their way somewhere—moving fast like all the cars. The highways are getting crowded here, but not so crowded as the coastal highways. Deep in the heart of the country there is still some privacy. There is still a way to look the other way when needed. We do all the basic things here that people everywhere do, the basics being slightly more at the forefront of our minds. Not so far below there is still a vast and restless ground that we rarely penetrate, silent and mysterious like a dream.

In the dream this morning, after I read you the letter, you took my hand in yours and we walked. Somehow we made it back to the old red house that has been torn down for years. The porch was still slanted with an over-dry woodpile under the front window, and inside a cat was sleeping on an unmade bed in the back room. A few flies buzzed. The remains of a fire in the woodstove were still going, though, outside, the field along the house was full and green. It was there in the dream out in the field that you looked up at me with a face I recognized from a long time ago and said, just before I woke, what the poet Rilke wrote a long time ago in a letter to a friend: "Be happy about your growth, in which of course you can't take anyone with you, and be gentle with those who stay behind."

Yours,

Pieta Brown

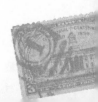

Donna Buell

Born in 1960, Donna Buell grew up on a farm in Ida County. She spent most childhood days outside with her cousins, father, and grandfather. Buell's family raised cattle, hogs, ducks, chickens, oats, alfalfa, corn, and soybeans. In 1979, she left Iowa to attend college in Florida, and lived in various cities in the southern U.S. until her eldest child entered kindergarten in 1995, at which point she returned to rural Iowa with her family. Buell practices law in Spirit Lake and serves on the Iowa Environmental Protection Commission.

Dear Young Iowan:

You know that Grant Wood painting, the one with the farmer and his daughter in front of their home? Now just put a big red "X" through it. No longer allowed. Grandpa is being driven out of his home. Your birthright is being taken from you.

After years of living in large cities in Florida and Texas, I moved back to rural Iowa. I wanted to be close to my family and especially to raise my young children on the land. I bought an old house on a lake close to my elderly parents, spent a lot of money fixing it up, found employment, and turned my kids loose with the dogs.

Soon afterwards, I discovered that a factory farm developer had purchased land upwind of my new country home. But the bigger shock was discovering that some of our Iowa legislators appeared to have sold us rural inhabitants right down the river.

Did you know that Iowa counties are currently prohibited by state law from zoning the siting of factory farms? Local communities have no say over where animal factories may or may not be built. And the protections our legislators have given us are laughable. Facilities can be placed as close as one quarter mile to your house. Manure can be spread right up to your property line. Every single rural home, business, and town is vulnerable.

Every pig makes ten pounds of excrement each day. Take that times thousands and sometimes tens of thousands of pigs, with all the excrement draining into a cesspool under the building and vented out with fans to prevent the pigs from being poisoned and dying—vented into the air with no regard as to who might be living, working, or having a birthday party 1251 feet downwind.

When the cesspool gets full, livestock sewage is spread on the land. Those days you gag just going outside, or driving down the road. The local river stinks and is slimy, black muck sticks to your feet when you wade in the water.

Who is left on the land in Iowa? Mostly the elderly are left—hard-working, independent, and now aged people struggling to maintain their health and independence. Many are farmers themselves, though they have no way to protect themselves from the new industrial agriculture.

Recently a couple from the next town came to call on me. The man, now elderly and a little shaky, proudly told me how he made it through the farm crisis of the 1980s with his family lands intact. Then he showed me a brochure for a factory farm corporation from North Carolina and a business card for the "site developer" who was buying the land one quarter mile upwind.

I couldn't help them. The best I could do was to explain about the tiny separation distances, the manure management plans, the matrix system, the non-role of the supervisors, and how quickly it will all move once the producer starts building. His wife, elderly too, had a notebook where she tried to scribble some notes, but the information I had to share was detailed, confusing, overwhelming.

Unfortunately, the conclusion was simple. "You are screwed," I told them. "There is nothing you can do to protect yourselves. My best advice is to sell out now while maybe you can still get something for your place." When they left, I cried.

Iowa's farmers are almost gone. There is no longer any way to make a decent living on the land. Farming has turned into agribusiness, and it does not take many people. Iowa residents are mostly urban now, and most jobs are industrial. The Iowa of my youth is almost gone.

Still, some of us try to hold onto rural life, onto small town life, although necessarily with new and different approaches. Might there be a way to get back at least some part of what we have lost? What about going back to raising food on the land rather than in factories? Maybe health-conscious consumers would be willing to pay more for that. What about rural tourism? If kids these days no longer have the option of going to grandma's farm, maybe their parents would pay to stay at a country inn where, for a few hours, they can pet a goat, see pigs and chickens roaming in a pasture, and romp free with their dog.

If you ever daydreamed of the country, now is the time to defend your state. Use the energy and smarts of your youth. Speak up. An Iowa without care for rural elders, without farmers, and without small towns will have lost its essence.

Sincerely,

Donna Buell

Tim Carman

Tim Carman's roots in Iowa extend back before the Civil War when his great-great-grandfather, Alpheus Carman, settled in Floyd County in 1858. After graduating from Hawkeye Community College in Waterloo in 1982, Carman attended Wichita State University in Kansas, and went on to a career as an engineer at Rockwell Collins in Cedar Rapids.

Tim Carman lives in Center Point in Linn County with his wife, Sandra, and their two teenagers, Megan and Brett. Their interests include biking on the Cedar Valley Nature Trail near their home and fishing the area's many lakes and ponds.

Dear Young Iowan:

At this stage of your life, you're no doubt asking: What type of work would I enjoy doing? What job would be the most rewarding? And an even farther-reaching question: How can I benefit my community and state by what I do for a living?

When most people think of vocations that help their fellow man, they typically think of medicine or social work or politics. Granted, these can be very noble professions, (though some would argue that point about politics), but I would like to propose an alternative—engineering.

I know what you're thinking: a greasy-haired, middle-aged man wearing high-water dress slacks, white socks with black shoes, nerdy glasses, and a short-sleeved, white dress shirt with a plastic pocket protector containing a half-dozen pens and pencils, and a slide rule.

I'm an engineer, and I haven't worn a white, short-sleeved dress shirt for some time now.

While engineering isn't often on the "A-list" for career choices, I can't think of a profession that has a greater potential for positively influencing your community, state, and world. While engineers may be retiring types, stop to think about all the ways engineers have made your life better, easier, safer, and more convenient—cell phones, microwaves, automobiles. The list goes on.

Iowa is not generally regarded as a high-technology state, and it is true that our heritage is largely agricultural. But did you know that one of the

Hawkeye State's largest employers is Rockwell Collins, a leading commercial and military aerospace company? Collins engineers design products that allow our armed forces to do their jobs more effectively and help air travelers fly with greater safety and convenience. The GPS technology found in many cars today was pioneered by Collins and the first words spoken from the moon by Neil Armstrong were transmitted by a Collins radio.

Need more examples? Consider the John Deere Company. Engineers there create products that help farmers in Iowa and elsewhere to produce more food to feed a hungry world.

Still not satisfied? Terex mobile cranes, designed in Iowa, are used all over the world for everything from helping to construct new buildings to removing debris for hurricane victims.

Engineering opportunities are not just limited to large Iowa companies, though. Small engineering firms abound in our state and produce a dizzying array of products from corrugated boxes to fabric solar panels.

Large companies or small, the engineers that work here in Iowa have one thing in common—they create products that solve a problem, make life easier, or help us do our jobs better.

Take a hard look at becoming an engineer, and imagine all the lives you could touch. And don't worry: we won't think less of you if you don't own a pocket protector.

Sincerely,

Tim Carman

Scott Cawelti

Scott Cawelti has taught film, writing, and literature courses at the University of Northern Iowa in Cedar Falls for thirty-eight years, and has written a regular opinion column for the Waterloo-Cedar Falls Courier *for twenty-eight years. He is now semi-retired, and with his wife, Angeleita Floyd, divides his time between Cedar Falls and Charleston, South Carolina, where he reads, writes, works on videos, and takes long walks on the Charleston Battery, with Fort Sumter always in sight. "We're fighting another Civil War," he insists, "only now it's between the Red and the Blue states rather than the Blue and the Gray."*

Dear Young Iowan:

Having grown up in Iowa myself some half-century ago, I sometimes feel like I landed on a different planet in 2006. Even though I still live mostly in Iowa, everything I do, see, and hear on a daily basis couldn't have been imagined by anyone growing up in Iowa five decades ago. A Fifties Iowan, suddenly transported in time, would feel utterly disoriented and alienated, less from time travel than from their first glance at the Internet and their (probably horrified) look at any HBO series. They would likely faint dead away or run screaming back to the safe and secure 1950s.

In my wildest teenage musings I couldn't have imagined cell phones, omniscient and omnipresent personal computers, the Internet, pervasive porn, video games, high-definition television images, global positioning systems, the demise of the family farm, "organic" food as a supermarket specialty item, expensive bottled water, voice recognition software, and anti-depressants and male impotence pills advertised on prime-time television. Or jet airplanes used as suicide missiles by religious fanatics.

Yet the vast majority of these changes have occurred in the last twenty years. And if one is to believe prognosticators such as Thomas Friedman or Ray Kurzweil even more radical changes will form our near future. The latter predicts in *The Age of Spiritual Machines* that within two decades, humans and machines will literally merge. Humans will sport a variety of computerized implants that will enhance and, in a sense, complete them.

Does that sound feasible? Probably not, but neither would the Internet have sounded feasible to a Fifties Iowan.

Some of you will revel in the changes, welcoming them with open arms and minds, while others will feel threatened, even horrified. Let me suggest that you would do well to revel in them, since you probably can't stop them, nor should you. Of course, anything from an unstoppable virus to massive climate change to a nuclear holocaust would interrupt all levels of technological and cultural change for decades, if not forever.

That in itself would bring catastrophic changes that we cannot imagine. Barring such horrors, humans will continue to seek technologies to enhance and improve their lives, often with unintended consequences. Distracted cell-phoning drivers making our highways more dangerous come to mind.

One piece of advice has helped me deal with such massive cultural and technological change, and it may help you. I read it years ago in an essay by novelist and nonfiction writer Norman Mailer: "Grow, or pay more for remaining the same." It struck me as wise advice then, and even more so now.

The temptation to stay the same, especially when "the same" is profitable, great fun, or just easier, can be overwhelming. In fact, some professions build in required "continuing education" credits to keep their colleagues abreast of recent developments. No one wants a doctor who's not aware of changes in treatment protocols or a teacher who hasn't kept learning and experimenting with new approaches.

Over the years, I have found two basic attitudes reside in those who resist and avoid change: traditionalism and obsessiveness. Traditionalists would keep the old ways going forever if they could. Or they simply fear the new technologies will harm them in some crucial way. The old-order Iowa Amish are a case in point; though admirable for their conservation and thrift, their nineteenth-century rural lives would not sustain our current urban culture.

Traditions are important, even crucial, but within a context of reasonable change. Family values can be maintained just as well in techno-wise families as techno-free ones.

Obsessed people are even more likely than traditionalists to resist change. One of the worst side effects of an obsession with, say, alcohol (or any high-inducing drug) is that it "freezes" emotional growth. If you become an alcoholic when you're eighteen, you stay eighteen mentally until you overcome your addiction. Only then can you grow out of the addiction into true adulthood with all of its opportunities and challenges. Anyone who knows an older, alcohol-obsessed adult realizes that they haven't changed much since they started drinking. In fact, they're probably worse, since they pay more for remaining the same.

So Mailer's advice is another way of saying "avoid becoming obsessed with anything to the point of addiction." Still, I do believe in following your passions. For years I've had a passion for the movies, with knowing about them, teaching them, even writing screenplays and editing videos. But it's all integrated into my life, part of a much larger group of activities that involves socializing, teaching, writing, and reading. And I've changed my mind dozens of times about the best approaches to making films, to teaching film, to film reviewing and criticism. Just bringing DVDs into film studies made me rethink everything I used to do with film before they were digitized.

Had I been obsessed with film, I probably would have been a "purist," insisting that film can only be studied on celluloid, that black-and-white films were artistically superior, that special effects are ruining film, and so on. People who were "addicted" to silent films resented "talkies" in the late 1920s, claiming they ruined film as an art form.

Finding a balance between a powerful, ongoing interest and addictive obsessiveness becomes a life challenge, as does finding a balance between maintaining traditions worth saving and those needing change.

Given the tidal wave of cultural and technological change that we all face in the near future, I try to live by Mailer's advice to grow, or pay more for remaining the same. But it's not easy.

Mike Chapman

A native of Waterloo, Mike Chapman has authored eighteen books, and his articles have appeared in a dozen national magazines. In April of 2002, he retired as publisher of the Newton Daily News, *ending a thirty-three-year career with newspapers. He was sports editor of* The Gazette *in Cedar Rapids from 1978 through 1984.*

Chapman has won numerous awards for journalism and writing, including the National Wrestling Writer of the Year (four times) and the Lifetime Achievement Award from the Cauliflower Alley Club, a national organization of former boxers and wrestlers. Along the way, he has interviewed such people as Muhammad Ali, Robert Redford, Lou Ferrigno (The Incredible Hulk from TV fame), and many other famous stars of movies and sports. Chapman is likewise something of a celebrity, having appeared on dozens of radio and TV shows, and having been featured in the TV show The Unreal Story of Professional Wrestling—*the highest-selling documentary ever produced by the A&E Network. Currently, he is the executive director of the International Wrestling Institute and Museum in Waterloo. His novel* GOTCH: An American Hero *is currently being considered for a major motion picture.*

Dear Frank Gotch:

It's a tremendous pleasure to write to you after decades of admiring you and all you accomplished during your lifetime. I am writing because I wanted to tell you what an enormous impact you have had on the sport of wrestling in general, and the state of Iowa in particular.

Not many wrestling fans realize how much they owe you, Frank. Nor do they know what a fascinating life you had, in and out of the ring. They would be surprised to discover that your parents immigrated to the United States from Germany while still in their teens, and that your father, Frederick, fought in the Civil War. Like many Union soldiers, he moved west after the end of the war, and he and his wife, Amelia, settled in a small village in northern Iowa named Humboldt.

Life was rough back then for the many Iowa families trying to carve out a meager living on a farm. There was plenty of work to be done by all nine

Good Sense from the Good Folks of Iowa

of the Gotch kids, and when your father's arm was crippled in an accident, you and your brothers had to absorb most of the work.

There was precious little time for schooling, but I know that was okay with you. You loved all sports, and your competitive nature really sprang to life when you engaged in local wrestling matches. I heard that you were always tussling with older boys because you loved a challenge and wanted to test yourself against bigger and stronger kids.

You established quite a reputation as a local wrestler, and when you met the great Farmer Burns, of Big Rock, Iowa, everything changed. Training under him made you the best in the world. Farmer was world champion years before he met you, and under his tutelage you really began to grow as a wrestler. The trip you took to Alaska in 1899, when you were just twenty-three years of age, really amazed me. Yes, you won all your matches and came back with nearly $30,000, but your friends in Humboldt had a mighty scare when they heard the boat you were scheduled to leave Skagway on sank, and all onboard drowned. Thank heaven you were delayed in getting to the dock and missed the boat, or the world would never have had Frank Gotch to cheer!

Your matches with American champion Tom Jenkins were so brutal that many fans were shocked. All of Iowa was proud when you whipped Tom and became the new heavyweight champion of the nation.

Then you beat the famous Russian Lion in Chicago on April 4, 1908, and became the new champion of the entire world. Half of Humboldt was on the town square waiting for the news to come over the telegraph wires. When it was announced that you had won, a huge bonfire roared into the night and the celebration went on till morning. The entire state was so proud of you, Frank.

You became pretty big stuff back then. I read that President Teddy Roosevelt invited you to the White House and you starred in a play that drew sold-out crowds in America and even Europe. Everybody wanted to be like you, Frank. You were the biggest hero Iowa had ever seen!

Your rematch with The Russian Lion in 1911 attracted thirty thousand fans to brand new Comiskey Park in Chicago. It was the largest crowd ever to see an athletic event in the nation's history, and hundreds of fans stood outside your hotel room the night before, hoping to see you. And you whipped him again.

The story about you marrying young Gladys Oestrich is so sweet. She tried to sell you a raffle ticket for the local church, and you told your friend that you would marry that gal someday. And marry her you did. Then you built her the nicest house in Humboldt. It still sits in the center of town, and you'd be shocked to know that fans still come to see it.

But life turned cruel, Frank, as we know it can. The news of your strange illness was shocking to everyone. No one could believe it when you lost so much weight. Humboldt people were so sad to hear that you could not even sit up in bed the last week. When you died, on December 17, 1917, the entire state went into mourning. Your passing made front-page news all over the country. Over two thousand people came to your funeral, Frank, and trudged along the path on a cold, wintry day to the cemetery to pay their respects.

I think you'd be pleased to know how important you are to the state of Iowa nearly one hundred years after your last match. Wrestling is a sport that demands hard work, sacrifice, dedication and determination. There is another very famous wrestler now, Dan Gable. He says that America needs wrestling because it teaches the same values that made America great.

I think you'd agree with Coach Gable, Frank. You two are a lot alike, in many ways. And you'd be proud to go to the state wrestling tournament in Des Moines and see the huge crowds. Fans come from all across the state to cheer for their schools and athletes. The tournament sells out in one day, and has been called the best high school state tournament in the entire nation, in any sport.

Wrestling has helped define Iowa and make it what it is today—a land of men and women who take immense pride in their work ethic and their devotion to duty. I have done lots of research on you, and know how proud you were to be an Iowan. When the big-city promoters tried to get you to move to Chicago or New York, you just shook your head, smiled, and said: "Fellas, I was born an Iowa farm boy, I was raised an Iowa farm boy, and I will die an Iowa farm boy."

You were much more than a great wrestler I have found out. You were a successful businessman who owned large portions of Iowa farmland, as well as an automobile dealership. You were generous with your support of charitable causes and loved being "just another man about town." I know you were being courted as a possible candidate for Governor in 1920, and that Hollywood was talking to you about starring in a movie when you got sick.

But uerimic poisoning and kidney malfunction changed all of that, Frank.

Recently, I drove past the old farm site where you grew up, and I could almost see you walking down the lane, a young man ready to challenge the entire world. I think you'd be pleased to know that Frank Gotch State Park is just south of your old farmstead.

I also drove past the house that you, your wife, Gladys, and young son, Frank Jr. lived in at the time of your death. And, of course, I drove out to Union Cemetery to pay my respects. I stood in front of the huge mausoleum that has the name *Gotch* carved at the top, said a prayer, and stared out across the Iowa farmland in the distance. I saw the waving fields of corn and felt the warm sun and a gentle breeze, an Iowa breeze.

I thought of how great an impact wrestling has had on Iowa, and what a great impact you have had on wrestling. I knew I was in a very special place at that moment.

I wanted you to know that you haven't been forgotten, Frank. Thank you for the legacy you have left to all Iowans. And thank you for never leaving for the bigger city, and remaining "an Iowa farm boy" all of your life.

Sincerely,

Mike Chapman

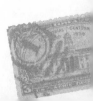

Hal S. Chase

Dr. Hal S. Chase was born in Des Moines, but spent ages eight to eighteen in segregated Frankfort, Kentucky. There he reports that the Civil War was still being fought, and that he was a "Yankee" or "Damn Yankee"—terms of derision because they were associated with sympathy towards African-Americans—to white classmates. Conversely, blacks, he writes, identified him as "white" except for his friend, John Sykes, who saw beyond the color of his skin.

Seeking "the inside" led Chase to degrees from Washington & Lee University (BA), Stanford (MA), and the University of Pennsylvania (PhD) and specialization and publication in African-American history. Chase teaches U.S., African-American, and Iowa History at Des Moines Area Community College-Urban Campus, and, since 1984, has served Farmers & Merchants State Bank of Winterset as a director and majority shareholder. He and his wife, Avril, a registered nurse, have four grown children and five grandchildren.

Dear Young Iowan:

One of the most overlooked and under-appreciated aspects of Iowa life is its rich African-American history. It's one you ought to know more about because you will live in an increasingly diverse state, nation, and world.

Through words and photographs, you will see that Iowa's African-American history is long, rich, and rewarding. You will also see that it is *our* history, a history of the inseparable, intertwined, intimate relationship between so-called "black" and "white" that lies at the heart and soul of Iowa and of the United States. Iowa's development is an integral part of the development of the western hemisphere in the last five hundred years that began with the transatlantic slave trade in 1502. It lasted for three hundred years and bound together the destinies of Europe, Africa, and the Americas. One major result was the rise of capitalism and global imperialism by Spain, England, France, and the United States. It was also the foundation of the industrial, urban, and commercial culture that dominates our time.

So it is fitting that an African-American was part of Iowa's history from its beginning. York, an enslaved man, was a member of the Lewis and Clark exploration of the Louisiana Purchase in 1804-06, which made Iowa part

Good Sense from the Good Folks of Iowa

of the U.S. It is equally fitting that the first case decided by our territorial Supreme Court was "the Case of Ralph," which outlawed slavery in Iowa in 1839. But Iowa, like other midwestern states, was not free of racial prejudice. Our first public schools were for "white" students only. But in 1868, eighty-six years before Brown versus State Board of Education, Topeka—which struck down separate schools for blacks and whites in 1954—Alexander Clark Sr. successfully sued the City of Muscatine so his daughter, Susan, could attend the white elementary school. This was the same year that Iowa became the first northern state to guarantee black men's right to vote.

No doubt you know about George Washington Carver and the role that Simpson College and Iowa State University played in his world-renowned career. But it is a good bet you haven't heard of Buxton, a company-owned coal mining community in southeast Iowa from 1900 to 1922, where the relationship between black and white was described by one resident as "a kind of heaven."

You also might not know that the first U.S. Black Officers Training Camp took place at Fort Des Moines during World War I, and that during World War II, it was the site of the first Women's Army Auxiliary Corps (WAAC) Training Camp. But these and other positive examples of our African-American history did not defeat white racism in our state. In 1948 Edna Griffin and others won their suit against Katz Drug Store in downtown Des Moines for refusing them ice cream cones.

You probably do know that the 1950s and 60s brought positive changes in the relationship of black and white Iowans and Americans. Examples of this include the election of the first black state legislators and the appointment of the first African-American judge. In the 1970s Cheryl Brown of Luther College became the first African-American to compete in the Miss America Pageant, Des Monies native and one-time Iowa middle school teacher James Harris won election as the first African-American president of the National Education Association, and Jimmy and Lou Porter founded the first African-American radio station, KBBG, in Waterloo.

The 80s saw more Iowa firsts, such as the election of the first black state senator (Thomas Mann, Democrat, Des Moines) and county supervisor (George Boykin, Democrat, Woodbury County), and the appointment of Dr. Percy Harris to the Board of Regents. The 90s brought even more:

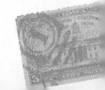

the first African-American mayors, sheriff, and state party co-chair (Leon Mosley, Republican, Waterloo). Yet, it was the miraculous delivery of the McCaughey septuplets in 1997 by Dr. Paula Mahone and Dr. Karen Drake that put the African-American history of Iowa on our nation's front pages.

So from York to Doctors Mahone and Drake, blacks and whites have been living, working, worshipping, and playing together in Iowa, and all of this is a significant part of who we are. The more you understand and appreciate this relationship, the better our future and yours will be.

Sincerely,

Hal

P.S. You can learn more about our African-American history by asking your school or public librarian for *Outside In: African-American History in Iowa, 1838-2000.*

Kris Clark

An editorial writer and columnist for the multi-generational, family-run newspaper the Tipton Conservative, *Kris Clark worked at the Dakota Plains Legal Services for nearly twenty years, directing the program's six offices from 1992-1998. A native of Tipton and a 1970 graduate of Tipton High, Clark stayed close to home for her higher education at the University of Iowa, where she earned an undergraduate degree and two graduate degrees—an MA in Journalism and a law degree. Kris Clark now shares the home she grew up in with her mother, Ruth Clark, who is also a well-loved columnist for the newspaper edited by Ruth's son Stuart.*

Dear Young Iowan:

Pasts are particular and pasts are shared, and nowhere is that fact more beautifully clear than in Iowa. More than anything I care about the past as it relates to the future, both of my family and of my community, Tipton.

It wasn't until I went to South Dakota, after I graduated from the University of Iowa College of Law and passed the Iowa Bar Exam in 1979, that I first began to realize how important Iowa was to me. At about that time, I went to work for a federally funded legal services program called Dakota Plains Legal Services, and spent just under twenty years working on two different Sioux Indian reservations in South Dakota. These two places, the Cheyenne River Sioux Reservation and the Rosebud Reservation, couldn't have been more different from my life growing up in Cedar County.

Through my mother's side of our family we have strong roots in Cedar County. Her great-grandparents, Frederick and Hannah Hunick Hinkhouse, came to Sugar Creek township in 1853. Both were born in Germany. Since then there's always been a Hinkhouse in that township, although my uncle John, who has no children, will be the last in our family. I bet your family will also experience many lasts in your generation, but I bet they'll enjoy many firsts as well. Experience both fully and your love of place will deepen beyond your imagining.

Life on the Cheyenne River in Eagle Butte, South Dakota and, later, on the Rosebud Reservation in Mission, South Dakota starkly contrasted with the bucolic life, as I began to view it, back in Tipton, where first my father then my brother Stuart ran the local newspaper, the *Tipton Conservative*.

I was really out on the prairie, one hundred miles northwest of the capital of Pierre, South Dakota, in a semiarid region where there were often more cattle and horses than people. Also the culture of the Sioux, still vital in South Dakota, was dramatically different from what I knew from eastern Iowa. For example, South Dakota ranchers weren't like the friendly Iowa farmers I'd grown up with. It took a lot longer to get to know them and, because I was a lawyer working with "the Indians," they were wary of me. It was understandable.

The biggest difference between Eagle Butte Mission and Tipton, Iowa was the people. Again, it was a different culture, including both members of the tribe and what we always referred to as all the "non-Indians"—the white ranchers and business people who either lived on or near the reservations. There was also a great deal of poverty where I lived in South Dakota, a stark contrast to home. The more I'd come and go, usually at least three times a year, the more I'd notice it.

As I've aged, what's become most important to me about Tipton, the county, and, really, all of Iowa, is that we preserve our past. To do that I've become active in our local Friends of Historic Preservation organization and the Cedar County Historical Society, which was begun in 1958. My grandfather, Elmer Hinkhouse, was one if its founders. Through these groups, and by what I can do through the newspaper, I want people to remember where we came from and what our forebears did for us.

My real love is historic preservation, and in this part of Iowa there's lots to cherish and preserve. Tipton's historic, nineteenth-century downtown, Century Farms, and buildings on the National Register of Historic Places are a passion for me, as they are for many others. As I see you growing up, I want you to have the same chance I had to walk among treasures, gaze on them on a soft summer night from a courthouse square and imagine what it was like where you stand over a century ago.

This area is a beautiful place. During our life together, I want us to do what we can to steward this heritage for those who will follow us in this small corner of Iowa. Iowans know the best farmers are stewards—so, too, are the best local historians, entrepreneurs, and newspapermen and women. I hope you will join us.

Sincerely,

Kris Clark

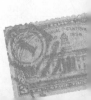

Dan Coffey

Dan Coffey is best known as public radio's purposefully pompous "Dr. Science." After receiving his Master of Fine Arts in Playwriting from the University of Iowa, Coffey and several friends journeyed to San Francisco, where they performed as the Duck's Breath Mystery Theater. Coffey returned to Iowa in 1988 to teach at the University of Iowa. He now teaches at William Penn University in Oskaloosa.

Dear Young Iowan:

If life were a theater experience, and I were casting a role called "Young Iowan," I would imagine a wholesome youngster in overalls, tanned from toiling in the fields, hard-working, naïve, sweet-natured, and civil. The male version would be in overalls; the female in a gingham print dress. Both would be well-acquainted with hard work, thrift, and church on Sunday.

This image is so clear because it's only a fantasy taken from movies and television. Unlike most viewers, I've been living and teaching in Iowa for almost twenty years now, and I know what real young Iowans look like. They wear tattoos and some have their tongues or noses pierced. They spend a lot more time playing video games than they do toiling in the fields. For that very reason, a good many are obese, and chugging down sixty-four-ounce soft drinks from the local Kum 'n Go has them courting diabetes.

So I'll picture someone like that when I give the following advice: get some sort of specialized training or you will be doomed to a life of poverty. By the time you're my age, fields will be cultivated, planted and plowed by remote-control, GPS combines guided by computer from Bangalore, India. All manufacturing jobs will have long ago gone to countries with lower standards of living. So it's going to become very black and white, very soon. Either you'll be living in a trailer on the edge of an abandoned town or you'll be able to live very well in this place with highly affordable real estate.

Learn Spanish. Most of your neighbors will speak it as a first language. If you want guaranteed employment, go into geriatric nursing, because there will be an endless need for workers to care for an aging populace.

Good Sense from the Good Folks of Iowa

If you make and implement the decisions to thrive, you will prosper and be able to usher Iowa into a new era of glory. Indeed, our state is behind the times, and that can be a good thing. We still have a lot of what used to be civil and sweet and shared by the other forty-nine states. Iowa is not yet a continuous strip mall full of franchised businesses. Iowans do not, as a rule, spend ten percent of their waking hours commuting to and from work. Most of our schools don't have armed guards and metal detectors greeting us at the front door.

So it's up to you. As you may have already noticed, an awful lot of young people leave for the Sunbelt as soon as they graduate from college. Those who remain until their children are grown, gravitate southward shortly thereafter. Check your local plat book and notice who owns the land around your town. You'll have a hard time locating many of those people in the local phone book. They're all in Phoenix, Dallas, and Orange County. That leaves you to stick it out here, capitalizing on our assets and tolerating our deficiencies.

I'll be here, too, I imagine. See you around.

Thomas Burnell Colbert

Born in Carroll, and a graduate of Scranton High School, Thomas Burnell Colbert has lived most of his life and done most of his schooling in Iowa, earning a BA and MA at the University of Iowa in 1969 and 1975 respectively before moving on to a PhD in History from Oklahoma State University, where his major topic of study was American Indian History. He is currently Professor of Social Sciences and Humanities at Marshalltown Community College, where he has taught American Indian history and Iowa history, among many other subjects, for twenty-five years.

Dear Young Iowan:

You might travel to the Meskwaki settlement near Tama and enjoy the yearly powwows or perhaps be entertained at the casino, but such activities are modern diversions and pale in comparison to the centuries-long history of Indian life in Iowa.

Indian peoples began to live in the area of Iowa about twelve thousand years ago, when they hunted now-extinct big game—mammoths and giant buffaloes. Around ten thousand years or so ago, natives began to make better stone tools in what became known as the Archaic period. Then, beginning about three thousand years ago, Woodland cultures began to emerge from the Archaic groups; people of the Woodland cultures hunted and gathered, made pottery, domesticated plants, and built burial mounds like those at Effigy Mounds National Monument in northeastern Iowa. The Indians of this time developed an extended trading network, importing valuable materials to be crafted into both usable and exquisite artifacts.

About one thousand years ago the Oneota culture spread throughout Iowa. No doubt related to later known tribes, the Oneota peoples lived in Iowa in decreasing numbers until about the year 1800. By then, other groups—contemporary tribes including the Winnebago, Potawatomi, Oto-Missouri, Yankton Sioux, Santee Sioux, Meskwaki, Sauk, and of course the Iowa—lived in Iowa. In all, it has been estimated that members of at least twenty historical tribes inhabited Iowa at one time or another.

Good Sense from the Good Folks of Iowa

Iowa has not always been a placid place. While many school children used to be told about the Spirit Lake Massacre, when several white settlers in northwestern Iowa were killed by angry Sioux in 1857, many of today's teachers seem to imply that Iowa escaped war and bloodshed on its own soil. The truth is more unpleasant.

Indian tribes fought viciously over hunting grounds, especially after around 1820, as whites pushed Indian groups westward onto other tribes' territories. Indeed, Meskwaki and Sauk conflicts with the Sioux were legendary. Eventually, the U.S. government signed treaties of removal with tribes in the state, mandating that the tribes leave by the early 1850s.

Still, many Meskwakis refused to relocate. They now considered Iowa their homeland, and their ties to the land outweighed any treaty their chiefs had signed. These dissidents hid out along the riverways until the Iowa legislature agreed to let the Meskwakis purchase land in Tama County. Today, the Meskwaki tribe is the only legally recognized tribe in Iowa, although members of other tribes reside in the state.

Iowa has a distinct Indian past. Having hunted for arrowheads, maybe, or done a scout or school project on American Indians, you know this much already. However, the state's Indian heritage is greater than its many Indian place names and designated historical sites. Likewise, Indian artifacts— from early stone tools to beautiful present-day beadwork displayed in museums across the state—only tell a part of the story.

An Indian presence is rooted in our past and our present. My injunction to you is this: recognize and appreciate our native predecessors and embrace a sense of *our*—Indian and non-Indian—mutual connection to Iowa.

Sincerely,

Tom

Shirley Damsgaard

Shirley Damsgaard's popular Ophelia and Abby mystery series debuted in August of 2005, and features the duo of town librarian and reluctant psychic, Ophelia Jensen, and her good witch granny, Abigail McDonald. Set in Iowa, the first novel of the series, Witch Way to Murder, *was nominated for an Agatha Award. The third book of the series is entitled* The Trouble With Witches. *Shirley lives with her family in Stuart, Iowa, where she has served as postmaster for the last twenty years. She is currently at work on the fourth book of the series,* Witch Hunt, *slated for release in 2007.*

Dear Young Iowan:

Have you ever been alone, on a gravel road—in the dark of the night, in the middle of summer? The hot air seems to hang around you like a shroud, and in the distance, trailing fingers of fog float across the road. Did you feel a bubble of fear form deep in the pit of your stomach?

Or maybe you and your friends have wandered around one of the old, abandoned farmhouses that litter our countryside. Did you imagine the voices of the past? The people who lived, loved, and died in those old houses? Did you have to fight the urge to run?

As a teenager growing up in Iowa, I experienced those things, too. I've told my share of ghost stories and been frightened by the late-night creaking of the old house I grew up in. I've hid under my covers, scared to move, knowing something lurked in my quiet bedroom, just waiting to pop out and grab me. My heart would thump against my ribs and my palms would grow clammy. The fear was real.

But as an adult I've learned it's not fear of things that go bump in the night that has the most impact on our lives. It's fear of failure, of being a fool. We all carry within us secret dreams that we never pursue because of those fears. We think about it, we imagine what our lives might be like if we had the courage to try, but in the end the bubble of fear, the urge to run, holds us back.

All of my life, I've dreamed of writing stories, but my fears stopped me. I thought my friends and family would laugh, think I was silly. Finally at the

Good Sense from the Good Folks of Iowa

age of forty-eight, someone whom I admire and respect encouraged me to set aside my fears and pursue my secret dream. And do you know what I discovered? My fears disappeared like mist chased away by the sun. No one laughed at me; no one thought I was silly. The worst thing that happened was I heard *no* from several publishers and agents, but eventually I heard *yes*. And all I needed was that one *yes* to make my dream a reality.

So I say to you, put your fear of failure in the closet, along with the ghosts, the boogeyman, and all those other imagined phantoms we fear. Trust me, nothing will leap out and pounce on you. Remember, the worst that can happen is someone might say *no*, but then again, they might say *yes*!

Live your life with courage.

All the best,

Shirley Damsgaard

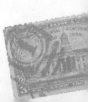

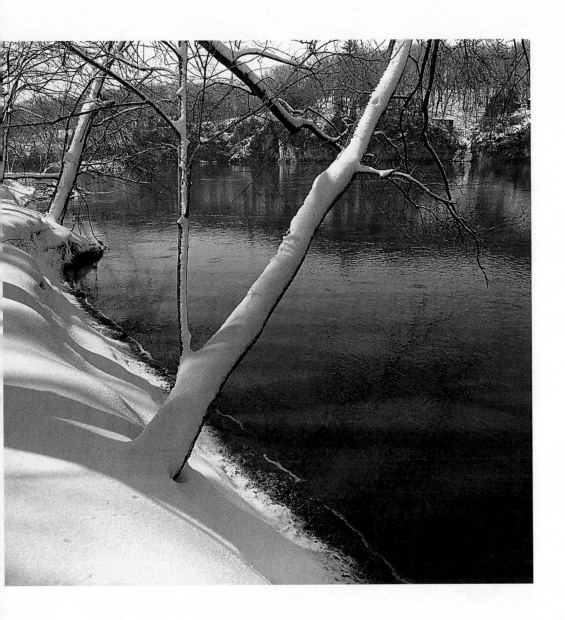

Photographs © Mark Petrick

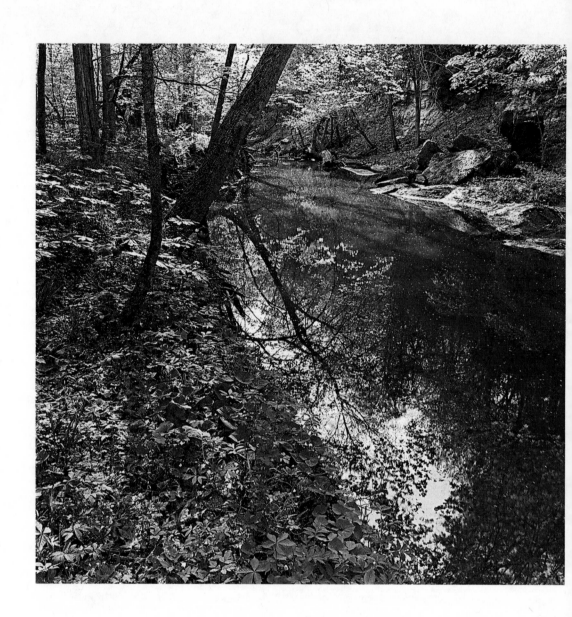

Les Deal

Five years after his birth in 1944, Les Deal and his family moved from Cedar Rapids to a farm near Anamosa, where Les attended a one-room schoolhouse. Deal went on to graduate with a teaching degree and a Masters from Truman State University. After five years of teaching, he opted out of the field in favor of the remodeling work that supported him through college and continues to support him today. In recent years, inspired by the power of his mother's poetry and his father's storytelling, Deal has become interested in the craft of writing. He credits his best-learned lessons in life to simple beginnings on the farm and in the one-room school.

Dear Young Iowan:

During my first year teaching school, I needed to experiment with soap-making. I wasn't about to risk doing the experiment for the first time in front of a class, so I went in on a Saturday. Sure enough, when I completed the experiment, I was convinced it had been a flop. I repeated it, carefully performing every step, only to fail again.

I couldn't understand it. I was trying to make beautiful, creamy soap, and all I got was scum floating on top. Finally it dawned on me not to expect a bar of soap with the word *DIAL* imprinted right on it. The "scum" was the soap!

I've been a remodeling contractor, by vocation, most of my adult life. Once, one of my long-term customers explained that he kept using me as contractor because on my first project for him—a balcony deck and an outside spiral staircase—I did everything he wanted and did it without resistance. In his eyes it was like a miracle. What he was saying was that I paid attention to what he wanted and made sure he got it. Said another way: paying close attention makes us better and wiser people.

I learned the power of observation as a child walking to and from school in rural Iowa. Our house was at the end of a mile-long dirt road, so my brothers and I learned to notice the difference in tire tracks and, often, could identify a visitor by the design of their tire tread. In the early spring, the roads would thaw during the day and freeze overnight, making it very hard and rough for the morning walk to school. It seemed every step we took alternated between the top of a ridge or the bottom of a rut. It made the going very tough.

Then I noticed something. The tiring part was stepping up and down, ridge to rut. I realized if I stayed up on top or down in the rut it required less energy. Even if I had to zigzag to stay on the same level it took far less energy to go back and forth on one level than to go up and down in a straight line.

Several decades later I was on a thirteen-mile, cross-country walk (no trail) with about forty others. About two-thirds of the way into the walk, one of the others said he had been watching how I walked and had been imitating my ways. In doing so, he was impressed how much easier it was and how much better he felt. I was using the same technique I learned on the dirt roads as a child. I was keeping my body as even as possible.

When you are in conversation, observe. Watch the eyes, listen to the words, and watch the body language. Each gives a message.

Once, in my late twenties, I was doing some work for a man and his wife who were both in their upper eighties. One day the elderly gentleman started telling me about his wife. He told me of a recent time when she got to the mailbox before him and hid the mail under the mattress. It took him two weeks to find his pension check. He continued telling other similar stories. Then he made a statement that hit me like a brick. He said she didn't even know who he was anymore.

Up until that moment I hadn't been looking at him. Up until that moment, I was hearing the words but failing to observe the depth of what he was saying. Tears flowed as he spoke.

In all our relationships we need to listen fully to get the most out of people and to put the most back into them. This is how we become caring, decent, and loving people.

As we pass through life, it is what we give from the heart that represents the best we have to offer. The depth and breadth of caring is caused by what you and I "feed" our hearts. It is not how many things we do in life that makes us grow; it is how much attention we pay to each thing we do that makes the difference.

Attentively,

Les

Thomas K. Dean

Dr. Thomas K. Dean is Special Assistant to the President at the University of Iowa, responsible for speechwriting, reports, and other writing and research. He also founded and directs the Iowa Project on Place Studies while holding an adjunct professorial position with the Literature, Science, and the Arts program at UI.

Known for his love of all things local, Dean has a regular place-based column in Iowa City's arts and culture monthly Little Village *and contributes creative nonfiction to a variety of Iowa-based publications, including* The Wapsipinicon Almanac, The Iowa Source, *and the Harvest Books Series volumes* Prairie Roots: Call of the Wild *(2001),* Living with Topsoil *(2004) and* Prairie Weather *(2005). His first book of essays,* Under A Midland Sky *is forthcoming from the Ice Cube Press, and he is also at work on a book about the wonders of the Minnesota North Woods. Dean lives in Iowa City with his wife, Susan Prepejchal, two children, Nathaniel and Sylvia, four greyhounds, two goldfish, and two cockatiels.*

Dear Young Iowan:

It's okay to love your hometown. It's okay to love Iowa. It's okay to love the Midwest.

I first knew a great love for home—in this case Iowa and Iowa City—when I left them. My heart ached for them. I felt an emptiness by their absence in my life. The sense of loss was not too unlike the physical and emotional feelings I experienced when my wife and I were apart during the year we were engaged because we were attending different schools, or the pain of absence I now feel for my entire family when I am away on a professional trip for even a couple of days. When I thought of Iowa after the years I left it—when pictures of the small spots that were meaningful to me entered my mind, when thoughts of past times walking by the Iowa River trundled into my reflection, when the unmistakable smell of Iowa summer humidity slapped my olfactory memory—the rush of warmth in my chest that I think we all understand as love was unmistakable.

Rather than dismissing these feelings as silly or simply nostalgic, I embraced them, even reveling in them. My willingness to let these feelings of love of place course through me had a lot to do with my determination—

and, happily, my success at—returning to the place I had come to know as home. So, again, it's okay to love home, Iowa, the Midwest.

The latter may sound like a silly or obvious statement. But, if you think about it, our society really encourages young people like you to feel that your hometown is restricting. We're told over and over again that we're a "mobile society," that the restless pioneer spirit is essential to our very character. You're a "success" only when you move up and out, to the big city, to the coasts, even out of the country. Staying put demonstrates a lack of ambition, or even failure.

The "get out" mentality is especially intense in the Midwest, and particularly so in small towns. Our fabled midwestern modesty often overflows into an inferiority complex. We are raised to believe that there's nothing special about the fields, the gentle topography, the plains, the "down-home" life of the middle lands. Our geographical flatness becomes a metaphor for life in the region. Certainly as individuals, as communities, and as a society as a whole, we're often stronger for the freedoms, economic success, and cultural understandings that come from the mobility we can enjoy. But there's a price to be paid when we sacrifice depth of experience in places we love for the breadth of a cosmopolitan ideal.

In an essay entitled "The Work of Local Culture," writer Wendell Berry reminds us that intergenerational continuity is the essence of community. He notes that the interruption of successive generations in one place, which has been the pattern of human history for centuries, undermines the passing of traditions that keep a place healthy and whole, and that keep us as individuals integrated socially and culturally. And Berry is also not afraid to talk about love when it comes to our home places. As he often says—especially in these times when community bonds are frayed, the uniqueness of our places is eroding, and our natural environment is suffering—we need to "give affection some standing." We do not misuse, let alone abuse or destroy, what we love, if we love rightly and well.

I don't think you really need an explanation for why it's important to love your home. But I suspect you would welcome permission to feel, to express, and to act upon those affections. I often teach college courses about the Midwest and its culture, as well as about the ideas of community and place. My classes often expose students to writers, thinkers, and other artists who love the Midwest and find great beauty in its fields, woods, towns, communities, horizons, skies, weather, plants, animals, rivers, and traditions. Many students are surprised by these expressions of love, often having never heard of anyone speaking positively about the midwestern landscape, small towns, or industrial cities, let alone affectionately. Our discussions, both in class and in one-on-one situations, often lead to what amount to student "confessions": that, really, they love their home communities and would like to stay there. But they feel pressured to think differently, by parents, teachers, peers, even the media and the culture at large. "You must leave home; otherwise, you are a failure." "There is no opportunity to grow in a small place." "Iowa is boring." "Get out while you can." "There's nothing to love here." Ironically, many of these people telegraphing such messages to young people like you are wringing their hands that the exodus they expect their own children to perform is exactly what is happening and that—surprise!—an awful lot of young people are leaving Iowa.

I realize there likely are economic factors impinging on your desire to stay home. I can't encourage you to do something that will harm your economic and life prospects. At the same time, I would encourage you to think about what you're willing to do for love. When you love another person, you get creative about making things work. I also understand that youth is the time of life to explore the world, to be open to new ways of thinking and living. So I'm not suggesting that you completely sacrifice your cosmopolitan impulses—they are healthy and should be acted upon, too. Being committed to a place for the long haul should not lead to insularity and ignorance. So go ahead and go away. Travel. Live somewhere else for awhile—or even forever, if that's really who you are. There will always be wanderers and explorers, and if you're one of them, you must answer the call of your identity. But remember that coming back home someday is a wonderful option, and you shouldn't feel ashamed of retiring your wanderlust when the time is right and settling down. You'll bring back new experiences and ideas that will refresh and revitalize your hometown. We need all of you—the wanderers, the returnees, the stayers. The main thing to honor is that love for home and the healthy desire to dig in.

So what gives you that warm feeling in your chest that I talked about earlier? Is it the sight of a verdant, dewy field of corn or prairie grasses

Good Sense from the Good Folks of Iowa

near your home on a cool summer morning? Is it the bonds of community you feel when you visit with friends and neighbors at a local café or coffee shop? Is it the sense of rootedness you feel after a satisfying dinner at your parents' house? Is it the Fourth of July traditions at your local park? Is it the simple beauty of the courthouse square or the bustle of your city's downtown nightlife? Whatever may give you that emotional rush of connectedness, realize that it is indeed love, that it's okay to feel it, and it's okay to act on it. Iowa deserves your love, and Iowa deserves your desire to stay home—or come back home someday—without apology. Some may say your ambition comes up short, but that's a mythology, not an absolute truth. Staying home or coming home because you want to commit to a place you love, and because you want to enlarge and deepen the sphere of community—through your work, your volunteerism, your love for place, and just living your life—are both great gifts and a magnificent way of life.

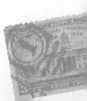

Mark Edwards

Mark Edwards graduated from high school in Sergeant Bluff, Iowa. Prior to his arrival in western Iowa, his family had spent three years with his Air Force father and family in Toyko, Japan. "When we arrived in western Iowa," he writes, "I buried my old self at the toes of the Loess Hills." Edwards attended Iowa State University and has lived on the Des Moines River ever since. He has worked as a trail coordinator for the Iowa Department of Natural Resources for twenty-five years, a position in which, he says, he is still learning the language of frogs and practicing what he calls "controlled folly." He dreams of being truly native to Iowa.

Dear Young Iowan:

When we were about your age, my friends and I used to walk to the bowling alley parking lot in the town of Sergeant Bluff. We hiked in a light drizzle across the flat field to the base of the Loess Hills. We knew of a cave behind the old brick factory that was our hideout. Circling around the small pond, we paused to make sure no one else saw us and then burrowed inside, out of the rain.

Every young Iowan needs such a place—a cave, a corner, a clubhouse.

The tunneled staircase penetrated deep into the Loess Hills and we kept climbing. We passed four rooms off of the main passageway. Each room could hold about four or five of us. There were low, flat benches like beds against some of the walls. Our flashlights further illuminated the sanctity of the place: names we didn't recognize, dates before we were born, and strange animal symbols decorating the vertical surfaces.

During other forays we would bring newcomers along, careful to approach the cave from the opposite direction to disorient them. We climbed the bluffs along the sloping ridge trail until we were almost at the summit. Then, with no warning, we ran ahead of the unsuspecting soul, dropping down a hole, disappearing like rabbits, leaving them to catch their breath and marvel at the magic of this place.

On special weekends we took sleeping bags to camp overnight on top of our world. Down in the town hazy, off-colored lights reminded us of

Good Sense from the Good Folks of Iowa

parents, teachers, and teenage resentments. We shared snickering and secondhand stories of sex for as long as our material would last—which wasn't long. We never exhausted our favorite fantasy of being Indians and men of the world.

We wondered if the cave was made by Indians, and if so, what they ate, and what they thought. Like the Indians, we resented interference from the outsiders invading our place. We were distracted by fast-moving cars we couldn't drive, screaming airplanes going somewhere else, and all the authority figures telling us what we could, should, and would do.

Sometimes we took those resentments out on each other by playing king-of-the-hill. We waited for the first person to fall asleep and then rolled them off the hilltop in their sleeping bag. You quickly learned not to zip up your bag and to keep your eyes open. Learning to dream while being half-awake made for visions filled with bison, birds, and rattlesnakes.

I've learned some things about loess since then that I want to share with you. Loess soils blanket two-thirds of Iowa and tens of thousands of square miles of the midwestern United States. It is the parent material of our nation's most productive agricultural soils. I was raised on it. I have been breathing and eating loess for most of my life. It's in my eyes, my blood, and my dreams.

In Iowa, ninety-four percent of our state's thirty-six million acres have been put to agricultural use. Roads and cities cover another five percent. Iowa is now known as the most biologically altered state in North America with over sixty percent covered in only two species, corn and beans. The largest part of the remaining one percent left undeveloped is in the Loess Hills.

What will we do? The question is not who owns the land and whether it remains private property or becomes a national park. The question is how we will, privately and publicly, live with it. Will we leave it undeveloped as an inheritance for future generations? Will we realize the little bit of wildness left in Iowa is part of our childhood, our education, and our community and spiritual life?

Why do we replace these soft, sculptured mounds with more flat, cold concrete? Why do we call the continuing destruction of the only small wildland pieces we have left development and progress?

We need these last oases of prairie remnants, of biological diversity, to be our legacy and remain as a monument to our maturity. We desperately need these wild places to show our children that we can make choices to have natural playgrounds, outdoor classrooms, and respect for God's creation.

Over the last forty years, I have stopped on numerous occasions traveling west to climb on Sergeant Bluff to the top of the world and have my visions. I love to lie in the prairie grasses and see where I have been, what's blooming, and where I am going. I like the clean feeling of loess on my skin like baby powder, the wind tickling my ears, and the earth in my eyes.

The view is majestic. Over the muddy Missouri River, a clear, deep-blue horizon sweeps off into the western plains. North lies Sioux City, a picturesque river town nestled into the hills. Eastward, the mounds have turned sharply from their normal north-south alignment and drift eastward in procession away from the river for miles. To the south the wide river basin teems with waterfowl and green growth.

My visions have become more rational with age. I now know there were elk, wolves, and grizzly bears roaming these hills. Last year I held a Clovis projectile point found near here and knew this was someone's home eight thousand years ago. I know the Indians dance and dream here yet today.

Last year I stopped again to touch base with my sacred spot. The cave was gone. The mountain was missing. Our beautiful bluff was carved up and carried away as cheap dirt in truckloads.

Once again I woke up shaken and bewildered, thrown off my hill. I hope you will be a more benevolent king than the usurping kings of late. And I hope you will come to western Iowa where your dreaming self can open up to grander hopes.

Dreamily,

Mark Edwards

Lori Erickson

Lori Erickson grew up on a farm in northeast Iowa and is a freelance writer in Iowa City. She is the author of Iowa: Off the Beaten Path *and* Sweet Corn & Sushi: The Story of Iowa & Yamanashi. *Her articles and essays have appeared in many regional and national magazines.*

Dear Young Iowan:

When I think about what it means to be an Iowan, here's the moment that comes to my mind. It happens at the end of each summer when my family and I are returning from our annual trip to the West. We are fortunate to be able to spend extended time amid the beauty of the Rocky Mountains and the immense vistas of the western Dakotas, but near the end of our long drive back home, there's always a joyful moment when I realize we're back in Iowa. It's usually evening by the time we enter the lush, rolling hills just east of Council Bluffs. After the dryness of the western plains, the Iowa landscape seems impossibly green and fertile, a rich, lush garden bursting with fecundity and bathed in the golden light of dusk. As we crest each rounded hill, I can feel my roots curl back into the soil of home.

That's my central image of my home state: Iowa as garden. That means we have less "wild" than many other places in the world, for ours is one of the most intensively cultivated states in the country. But we have rich soil here for nurturing life, whether you're a soybean seed or a human being. Those roots give Iowans a sense that we are part of a larger story, one that links the past and the future and that ties us to our fellow citizens.

Even in Iowa City, a community that has a higher percentage of transient folks than many parts of Iowa, one can feel those ties. They were vividly evidenced during the tornado of 2006, when a wide swath of the city was destroyed. In the days that followed, I was amazed at the industriousness and community spirit shown by countless people. Within hours of the storm, the clean-up began. Volunteers showed up in droves to help pick up debris. Many opened their homes to those with no home left to return to. In other parts of the world such acts of generosity would be considered extraordinary, but in Iowa they are routine. Because our roots are healthy here, we are strong enough to help others.

So my advice to you as a young Iowan is this: if you want to fly (as most young creatures do), you need to make sure your roots go deep. That may sound contradictory, but I think those two impulses are related. Too often we do one or the other. We think that to be adventurous and free means that one can't be tied to a community or place. Or we make the opposite mistake of mistaking fearfulness for roots, glorifying our inertia because we dream too small.

You can do both in Iowa. You can love the land, the people, and the traditions of this place. You can nurture connections with others in your community and work to save the natural resources that sustain us all. And you can still dream big dreams and meet the larger world with keen curiosity and zest.

As a freelance writer for more than twenty years, I've been fortunate to travel around the world for my work. I love the exotic cultures of foreign lands and the diverse beauties of other regions of the country, but part of what makes me enjoy my work is the rootedness of being an Iowan. When I land at our local airport after a long trip or cross the border of our state after an extended journey, I feel those roots grounding me. Sometimes the land is bathed in the golden light of a summer evening, and sometimes it's locked in the arctic grip of a January cold snap. But no matter what the weather, Iowa is still a garden to me.

It can be your garden, too.

Good Sense from the Good Folks of Iowa

Bob Everhart

Bob Everhart has been president of the National Traditional Country Music Association since 1976, and has performed old-time traditional country, folk, bluegrass, and prairie roots music in the United States and Europe for the past fifty years, recording six LPs for the prestigious Smithsonian Folkways label and earning a Grammy nomination in the process. Everhart's influence is international in scope, including three LPs re-released on foreign labels as well as numerous first-time releases in Ireland, the Czech Republic, Poland, and Germany. In Iowa, Everhart is perhaps best known for hosting the long-running Iowa Public Television show Old Time Country Music. *He is currently working on a new television show entitled* Bus Stop *that utilizes traditional music, arts, crafts, and travel features.*

Dear Young Iowan:

As president of the National Traditional Country Music Association, I write to you about the importance of music.

Country music as we know it today contains elements of every other kind of music; some of it you like, some of it you don't. The really different music I represent is the music of the soil, the music that came to Iowa in covered wagons, perhaps music played by your own ancestors as they settled this incredibly fertile and productive state. The music they played was pretty much homemade. They had only a few musical instruments—the guitar, fiddle, harmonica, maybe an accordion.

We don't hear those instruments much in today's "country" music do we? But, in our great state of Iowa, we still hear them a lot, especially as played by those traditional families that have instilled a strong desire in their own young people to carry on the genre. These "students" learn how to play old-time musical instruments by ear. That means they learn to play without the ability to "read" music, or follow a melody line of notes. Rather, they have a strong inner desire to play incredibly beautiful and inspiring music by simply listening to it, and passing it along to sons and daughters, nieces and nephews, neighbors and friends. Sometimes they do this from their back porch, never realizing how really good they are. They don't seek fame or fortune. What they do seek is excellence in playing the music of our pioneers and forefathers—the simple but beautiful expression of our collective positive feelings.

Music is a wonderful pursuit. It can be one of the most satisfying adventures in a young person's life. It can take you to new places and new experiences you would otherwise never have had the opportunity to experience. It can place you in the role of "entertainer" for friends, family, neighbors, even strangers.

The National Traditional Country Music Association is made up of many people with like-minded ideals—so many, in fact, that we host an annual festival of old-time music now in its thirty-first year. So the reason for this letter, finally, is to invite you to attend this remarkable event. Find out for yourself what old-time music is all about.

Timothy Fay

Timothy Fay operates a printing and publishing business, the Route 3 Press, on his family's Century Farm north of Anamosa. There, since 1988, he has published an annual letterpress edition of the Wapsipinicon Almanac, *a collection of essays, fiction and reviews.*

A 1975 graduate of the University of Montana at Missoula, Fay returned to Iowa after college and began collecting printing equipment after being inspired by Bonnie O'Connell at the Penumbra Press in Lisbon, Iowa and by his late uncle, Lewis Fay, a former compositor and pressman at the Anamosa Eureka. *For fun, Fay reports, he gardens, "monkeys around" on the farm, and plays mandolin in the Celtic band Wren. His adult children, Kate and Lee, have, he says, wandered to New York City and Steamboat Springs, Colorado, respectively.*

Dear Young Iowan:

Let's make these acres wild again! Straight, clean, endless rows of corn and soybeans are pleasant and a key to Iowa's economy, but there's too much order and conformity in the Iowa countryside. I'm all for turning this farm into a swaying sea of colors—a chirping, croaking, humming, growling chorus of wildlife—an always-being-tinkered-with work-in-progress. I'm hoping you're interested.

You are the youngest of the six children raised in this generation on these hundred acres in Cass township near Anamosa. I'm writing to you because you're the last child still residing here and you, at only eleven, are by far the youngest offspring. But I'm addressing you, too, because I've noticed your interests appear to lie pretty close to home. I know you love the wild, secret places on this little farm. Your dad has pointed out your forts, your fire rings, and your stone circles. I've never known a child like you who could entertain herself for hours so contentedly.

I'm proud to say that our two households have tried a few new things during the past thirty years. Your dad and I inherited this place from your great uncle, who inherited it from his father, whose own father, an Irish immigrant, had passed it on to him. When your great-great-grandfather began working this land in 1863, wolves still roamed the township. Marshes no doubt dotted this farm as well as most others for all the three miles into town. An incredibly diverse cycle of wildlife flourished then. The steel plow, barbed wire and clay field tiles were beginning to corral the landscape and eliminate habitat, but hundreds of species of plants, insects, birds, amphibians, fish and mammals were only beginning their slow decline.

When I moved here in 1975, the then eighty-acre farm was almost entirely cultivated. My uncle had insisted his renters farm a rotation of oats, hay and corn, but the softly rolling landscape offered very little diversity. Serious wildlife cover was almost nonexistent. Your dad farmed organically for almost twenty-five years; his dairy and then beef herds took up residence but have since moved on. We rented the farm to neighbors two years ago, thus ending the organic experiment, but I must say that perhaps the real fun is just beginning, and here is where I must ask for your help.

I began planting many kinds of trees, shrubs, vines and groundcovers around my house many years ago. The birds liked that idea. At first it seemed only starlings and English sparrows frequented our surroundings. Now many songbirds call this home. Their music and colors brighten these acres, as they will continue to do if you keep planting and keep those feeders full.

Over the years we acquired the bankrupt railroad holdings through the length of the farm. That's become a delightful little nature trail. Throughout that stretch (where you've built your hideaways) you'll find different habitats: dry prairie, swampy stuff, mature hardwood stretches, and hearty mixes of all the above. Somebody, someday will have to keep the trail cleared. Those elms out there keep dying, and it doesn't take much of a windstorm to topple them. I'm going to keep whacking on those clusters of box elder trees to replace them with little white pines, walnuts, oaks, and hazel brush. But trees will need planting and care long after I'm gone.

You helped us clear ground for that wetland we're creating near the main road. I'm hoping you'll keep an eye on that, over the years, to insure our hoped-for population of salamanders, frogs, turtles, and new birds stay happy. The snipes, rails, and woodcocks are gone, but maybe they'll return.

Our current seventy acres of cropland doesn't need to stay that way. The Federal government is quite helpful in assisting in the removal of farmland from "production." Its cost-share programs encourage wetlands and wildlife cover. We put four acres this spring into native, short-grass quail cover, and Uncle Sam is paying us a fair rent to do it.

Someday we'll finish that humble little cabin on the north end of the farm—up there where you can't see a road or a brightly lit residence, up there where the windsongs, the birdsongs, and a screeching hawk or a deer crashing through underbrush is about all you're likely to hear. Perhaps that corner of heaven will be your occasional refuge from our zany civilization. You and your children can follow bluebirds there on a warm June morning or gaze at Orion on a ghastly-clear January night. The snow drifts may cover all those wild pleasures that evening, but as you slip another log into the cabin's stove, you'll know that spring, with its awakening smells, sounds, and sensations, is only a heartbeat away.

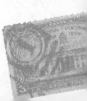

Hugh Ferrer

After earning a degree in philosophy from Princeton University in 1990, Hugh Ferrer worked in New Orleans, Boston, the mountains of upstate New York, Europe, and the Middle East. While attending the Iowa Writers' Workshop, Hugh and his soon-to-be wife Jane lived in Swisher. After he received his MFA in fiction, they began a family and moved to Iowa City, where they are now raising their two children, Callum and Sophie. Ferrer joined the staff at the University of Iowa's International Writing Program in 2001. He is now Associate Director of the IWP and the fiction editor for The Iowa Review.

Dear Young Iowan:

It is early afternoon in Iowa City and around midnight in Baghdad. The neighborhood leaders have wheeled wooden carts to the end of their streets and erected the barricades they will man all night in an attempt to keep out the death squads now marauding the city. The long-incipient, Sunni-Shia civil war has begun in earnest. We have lit a match in a fireworks warehouse.

Most of your life will transpire in the shadow of this war, its fears and enmities, its necessities, its dictates—its absurdities and rapes, its love stories, its moments of bleak serendipity ... its interpretation and re-interpretation. "Where were you on 9/11?" will be a password question to which you, only a few months old at the time, will always lack a good answer, just as I always lacked an answer to "Where were you when Kennedy was shot?"

It's hard to put into words the national sea change that followed, but I want you to know: this country was a less fearful place before. Since 9/11 we have been led towards anxiety by those who should have been exciting our courage. In our panic and need for retribution, in the cold shadow of our vulnerability, we sanctioned two wars—one in Afghanistan and a second in Iraq. Almost five years later, we are still in a wartime state of mind. The country has become more polarized, the major parties are at each other's throats; detractors of the president are called "traitors" and accused of "helping terrorists."

Good Sense from the Good Folks of Iowa

Local life in Iowa City has not changed terribly much due to the "War on Terror." The building of Coral Ridge Mall had a far more tangible impact on the city's fabric. There are no random searches on University buses, but there are new layers of fear guiding everyone's small habits. In a hallway or on a bus, people now view an untended bag or a piece of left luggage with at least some concern. I would guess that Iowa City's Muslim citizens and "Arabic"-looking citizens have felt discomforting and alienating suspicions directed at them.

The most obvious physical changes occurred at our closest "border," the Cedar Rapids airport, where big screening machines hulk beside the ticket counters and where you now kiss hello or good-bye outside security. There are padded chairs to sit on as you wedge your shoes back on. There are random searches conducted by polite, good-natured, often burly security guards. For a while, when the national, color-coded security level rose, airport security set up a checkpoint away from the terminal and inspected cars' trunks. Add up all the security and you must leave for the airport half an hour earlier than before. Everyone accepts these changes—anything to feel safe on a plane.

I recognize the fear in myself by the addiction to Internet news I've developed since those events; the paper arrives on our doorstep, but most of it seems a day late.

And then, of course, military personnel have been mobilized, mostly young volunteers, plus National Guard units and ROTC students, almost all what Louis-Ferdinand Céline called "virgins to the horror." I don't believe anyone from Iowa City has been killed in Iraq yet, but nearby towns and cities—Tipton, West Liberty, Cedar Rapids, Anamosa, Mechanicsville—have each lost a son. Veterans in their young twenties are returning to college classes, divided from their classmates by the experience of war; vets who have adjusted are helping those who haven't.

In light of these changes, some advice: To the extent that our leaders, our news shows, and our culture promote fear and paranoia, look for courage and moral leadership elsewhere. Try to embrace FDR's "firm belief that the only thing we have to fear is fear itself—nameless, unreasoning, unjustified terror which paralyzes needed efforts to convert retreat into advance." (Henry David Thoreau is just as good: "Nothing is so much to be feared as fear.") Please rejoice in American individualism, our communal holding aloft of personal ingenuity: the belief, recognized as early as Alexis de Tocqueville, that each of us can judge things for ourselves. But you must balance it wisely, maturely, with that ghostly part in each of us that binds us one to another—to our families and neighbors, and to even larger groups. I'm talking about that part that is not *me*, but, rather, *we*: the often dangerous, collective part of our identities. In some crowds, then, keep your head; in others, go ahead and lose it!

The world will not leave us alone here. It is woven more tightly than that. I don't know how the various military campaigns will first touch you. A video game? A recruiter at City High School? A friend's brother KIA? A convoy from the National Guard base on Benton Street in the University of Iowa homecoming parade? But touch you they will, and I worry about how you and your friends will deal with the call to "vigilance" and the assertion of ubiquitous "enemies."

Will patriotism be a collective *we* for you? What will "we Americans" mean to you? Will you feel called to duty? What role will fear play? Will the political polarizations and extended war efforts demonize not signing up? Through all of this turmoil, I hope you will use your tremendous imagination to create a *we*, finding at least one small shared element with the enemy, whoever the enemy is that day. People are more alike than they are different.

(I feel the speed of culture already pushing us apart. Young Iowan, how hard you and I will both have to work if we're to hold anything in common...)

While I have been composing this letter to you, a young man came to the door. From where I'm sitting, I could watch him cross the street, adjust his clipboard, assess how friendly our dog, waiting and wagging at the screen door, was going to be. His security company, a conglomerate of Honeywell and another company, has been seeking houses "to help out." Several houses over there, he said, pointing towards the cemetery, have agreed to help— and he showed me a list of names. Did I know them? I didn't. Anyway, he said, in this neighborhood, "one or two houses" was all he needed. For displaying the company's oval sign in our window ("Protected by Security System"), we would get a security system installed, plus fire and medical insurance. I said we didn't need a security system, that we live here in part because we don't. Yes, he nodded, that's what others—here he gestured vaguely towards Happy Hollow Park and down Brown Street—had said, that it's really a nice place to live. He listened politely as I responded with Jane Jacobs' theory—that a street becomes safe through the steady gazes of those who live there. He didn't point out, bless him, that a security camera or a drone might have been as effective.

I wished later that I'd lied to him about who nearby rented, and who was an owner. I shouldn't have made it easier for him to place in anybody's window the suggestion that the rest of us are "unprotected" and less safe than our prudent neighbor. It's a pernicious business, selling security.

I don't think I can imagine a starker contrast: on the one hand, a quiet residential street in Iowa City—a resident turning down a free security system—and on the other, a long, frightening night spent atop wooden carts, a neighborhood militia warding away roving opposition death squads. But they are connected, now. Not as in the government slogan—we must fight them there, so that we don't have to fight them here ("here" never meant Iowa.). They are connected because a fight everywhere now—not the only fight, but an important one—will be with fear itself.

I hope together, in this gentle place, we can preserve and pass on at least some small sense of peace.

Yours affectionately,

Hugh

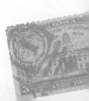

Mary Flagel

Mary Flagel is a first grade teacher in Maquoketa, Iowa, where she brings thirty-five years of teaching experience to her students. Widowed, she has one son, two grandsons and one step-granddaughter.

Dear Young Iowan:

I was raised on a small farm in Iowa. I lived on the farm from the time I was five years old until I left the farm to go and seek my fortune as a teacher when I was twenty-one.

Through the years I learned many things from the animals on the farm.

From the cattle I learned that you can indeed get too much of a good thing. If cows get frisky and jump a fence to get into a clover field on a summer day, they can "bloat." Bloating is a special condition caused in cattle when they eat too much clover, causing all kinds of distress as gasses are released into their seven stomachs.

I also learned that cattle, like people, have a special rule: "Everything looks better on the other side of the fence." They will crowd and push on a fence to get grass, to get water, to see another cow or, just out of curiosity, to check out something new.

Cattle have a social order. They push other cattle away from the feed bunk. Sometimes they will fight. If one cow leads, other cows will follow (even if they do not know where they are going or what they are going to do when they get there). They kind of remind you of politicians at a political convention.

Cattle have family problems similar to humans whose children grow more independent. Cows and their calves will bawl for days when separated at weaning time. It reminds you of the separation anxiety felt by kids on the first day of kindergarten, first day of college, or when they get married.

Pigs, on the other hand, have very little personality or drive. Their only goal is to find something to eat, and to find someplace where they can wallow in the mud and sleep. I have met some men who have similar goals.

Poultry are a lot like some families. The roosters strut around the barnyard all day crowing, showing off and fighting. The hens work their tails off finding food, laying eggs, and raising the baby chicks.

Did you know, however, that farm animals lead a dangerous life? Where else are you fed and watered and treated so well only to be butchered and become Sunday dinner?

Our butchering involved chickens and usually took place in the late summer or early fall. The young hens were safe. They would molt through the winter and lay eggs in the spring. Most of the young roosters never did realize what was happening to them until they were put in the wooden crates while my dad went to get the sharpened ax or hatchet. It was like an assembly line after that.

My dad would kill the young roosters. And, yes, decapitated chickens do jump around like chickens with their heads chopped off. Then he would gut them and scald them in boiling water.

The next step in the assembly line was to pull off the feathers. It always amazed me how easily the feathers came off after the chickens were put in the scalding hot water. After the feather plucking the chickens were immersed in cold water. The next person, usually my mom, would cut the chickens into parts. It was a proud day on the assembly line when you were elevated to the position of cutting up the chicken. I still remember the day when I held that position. The last step was to freeze the chickens whole or cut-up to be used for winter food and sometimes sold to family and friends.

No farm would be complete without cats. The outdoor cats caught the mice and knew how to survive. The indoor cats, on the other hand, were a lot like movie stars. The indoor cats were self-centered with many ego problems. Their problems would occur if they were ever demoted and had to go outside. The reality of existence in the real would was often too much for them.

Probably the most trusted animal on the farm was the farm dog. I remember Shep, Dusty, Queenie, Goldie, Red Dog and Teddy. They would be watchdog, working dog (chasing cows), and constant friend to everybody. They each had a special burial spot on the farm when they died.

Growing up on a small farm meant experiences that were unique to that time. It was a good life even though it was not always a profitable one. My dad worked at a factory in town to make ends meet on the farm. My mom often took over the chores and field work when he was at work. They were remarkable people in how hard they worked on that farm.

I had wonderful parents. They encouraged us to do well in school and taught us the value of a hard day's work on the farm. I still remember unloading hay onto an elevator that sent the hay up into the barn where my brothers stacked it. Sometimes we would find a snake that had been baled into the hay. The iced tea and lemonade always tasted good after that job.

We also had fun on the farm. We had 4-H projects and 4-H camp, baseball games, fishing trips, ice cream socials, swimming parties, and the county fair in the summer. In the winter we went sledding and went ice skating on the creek.

The days of the small farms are decreasing. They are being replaced by large corporations with hog confinements and giant poultry farms where the chickens never see grass. There are cattle producers that handle the entire cattle industry—from the farm, to the slaughtering houses, to the grocery store.

Maybe I lived a segment of small farm history that may disappear someday. I hope not.

Sincerely,

Mary Flagel

Susan Futrell

Susan Futrell is a freelance writer who reports that she loves food, farms, farmers' markets, and books. Futrell worked in food marketing and distribution for twenty-five years and now provides communications, marketing, and research on food and sustainable agriculture through her company, One Backyard. In keeping with those interests, her current project is writing about heirloom apple orchards. She has a BS in Geography and an MFA in Nonfiction Writing from the University of Iowa. She was born in Iowa and lives in Iowa City with her husband, two cats, and a very small garden.

Dear Young Iowan:

One of the things I love most about being from Iowa is that it's easy to grow up knowing where food comes from.

By the time you grow up, the food you eat and the landscape you see when you drive across Iowa may be very different from what they are now—already they've changed a lot since I was a little girl. Maybe you will still see corn and soybean fields stretching far in many parts of the state. Most of the empty old barns and farmhouses that sit tilting with broken windows and weather-faded boards will be covered over, but who knows whether they will be covered with new houses and garages, or orchards and gardens. Maybe there will be fewer of the open vistas that Iowa is famous for now, and in their place will be more and more towns, every few miles, with houses and streets and gas stations and shopping malls and schools. Or maybe there will be more farms dotting the horizon, with windmills in long rows and vineyards, apple trees, greenhouses, potato and onion fields, beehives, and raspberry bushes making the view look like the multi-colored drawings you used to do at school and which we older Iowans gladly hung on our refrigerators.

Here are the kinds of things I hope you have a chance to know, growing up in Iowa.

Ripe, sour red cherries taste best sitting in an old cherry tree in the backyard, so high you can see the next street over, the limbs of the tree gnarled into a perfect, butt-shaped dip where you can pluck cherry after cherry for hours and hours without anyone knowing for sure you are there. A well-made pie from those same cherries can taste almost that good. Almost.

The best way to eat a Muscatine melon is when it is deep orange, mushy in the middle, and still warm from the back of the pick-up parked at the corner down the road, cut into a wedge and sprinkled with just a little salt. Forget the spoon and let it drip right down your chin.

To make grape jelly, pick the concord grapes in the backyard when they have turned a deep, dusty purple, and after they are cooked to mush, push them through a strainer so the juice runs out thick and clear. Top each jar with paraffin wax and slather on a sandwich in the middle of winter.

Fresh eggs feel warm and scratchy with straw and fit perfectly into the palm of your hand when you lift them like glowing moons in the dim light of the chicken coop. Hold gingerly, but almost tight, so you can get away fast from the cranky, bobble-headed, fluffy-yet-menacing hens.

Squirrel tastes like chicken. Thanks to Grandma Augustine, who made it and showed us that eating could be an act of bravery, a badge of honor as well as a good story.

For Sunday dinner of Aunt Laura's chicken and homemade noodles, the right amount of water to mix into the flour for the noodle dough is half an eggshell full.

Milk fresh from the cow is warm, not cold—and Uncle Donald really could squirt it right into the yellow barn cat's mouth. Whipped cream made from that milk thickens so fast, even with a hand beater, it turns into butter when you're not watching, which means fresh butter on crackers for lunch.

When the voice of the noon market report on the radio says "pork belly futures up," it is not a joke.

I know your mother loves to cook and that your garden is full of ripe tomatoes in summer. You know what good food tastes like. Here's one more thing I hope you know: to have food—real food, good food—you have to have farms.

It's easy to grow up in Iowa knowing where food comes from, but it's also easy to forget what you once knew. Remember with each sweet, juicy, adventurous, comforting bite.

May you love growing up in Iowa that much.

Love,

Aunt Susan

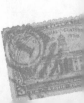

Dan Gable

Combined, Dan Gable's high school and college wrestling record at West Waterloo and Iowa State University respectively was a remarkable 182 wins and 1 loss, with the sole loss coming in his final NCAA match. After college, Gable, a Waterloo native, won World and Olympic championships, including an almost unbelievable gold medal run in the 1972 Munich, Germany Olympic matches in which his opponents went scoreless against him.

Gable coached at the University of Iowa for twenty-one years, winning an unprecedented twenty-one straight Big 10 titles and fifteen NCAA team championships. His record earned him the position of head wrestling coach for the Olympic games in 1980, 1984, and 2000. Dan Gable and his wife, Kathy, have four daughters, Jenni, Annie, Molly and Mackenzie.

Dear Young Iowan:

It's always great to know a little history in your home state, especially because it's nice to have people around you at least thinking you are well-educated about the past and looking to make a contribution to the future.

Let me get directly to my points. First, throughout the world, the state of Iowa is known for feeding global populations with our agriculture. In fact, a Nobel Peace Prize winner from Cresco, Iowa, Norman Borlaug, created a process for helping make food available around the world, especially in underdeveloped countries. He is credited with saving a billion people from starvation. Now *that* is important. Go anywhere in the world and mention the state of Iowa, and they know us for this important survival resource: food!

My second point is not as important to survival, but it too has spread throughout the world. And in one hundred and forty-three countries its characteristics develop leadership skills within families and societies. To help keep America's freedom, even the United States military looks for recruits with these same leadership qualities. I'm talking about the history—past, current, and future—of the sport of wrestling and its global effect. For over one hundred years, starting with world wrestling champion and

Good Sense from the Good Folks of Iowa

native Iowan Frank Gotch, Iowa has had World and Olympic wrestling champions that have helped keep our state's great name in the news.

To reiterate: one can go to the far corners of the world and mention Iowa and people know Iowa for good farming and good wrestling. Between the University of Iowa and Iowa State University, the state has had ten Olympic wrestling champions. And guess what? Even Norman Borlaug was a wrestler.

It makes sense!

Sincerely,

Dan Gable

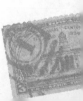

Lois Swartzendruber Gugel

Lois Swartzendruber Gugel was born and raised near Kalona. She taught elementary school for thirty-eight years, mostly in Johnson and Washington counties, but also in Newfoundland and Northern Alberta. She is currently working as an archivist in the Mennonite Museum in Kalona.

Dear Young Iowan:

It was a chilly November morning when you entered my fifth grade classroom in Kalona years ago. You had just moved here from Bosnia, and you learned English very quickly. In fact, you learned everything quickly, and your curiosity sparked our classroom.

Because we were in a public school, we didn't talk much about religion. When you asked me where I went to church, I told you I was a Mennonite and hoped that would suffice. Of course you wanted to know what that meant. I told you that Mennonites believe we should follow Jesus' teachings as taught in the Bible. Also that we believe our young people should not go to war and that we should not be baptized until we have made a commitment to follow Jesus. You seemed satisfied with the answer, and we went on about our schoolwork.

Now that you are nearly old enough to register with the draft board, I thought you might be interested in knowing more about why Mennonites in Iowa and elsewhere believe so strongly in nonresistance.

You may be wondering how my family has dealt with not serving in the military. Way back in World War I, my dad was drafted into the Army and went to camp as a conscientious objector (CO). He was mistreated by the officers and had to do the most undesirable work. But he was not sent to a battlefield.

In World War II, so many Mennonites were COs that the government provided a Civilian Public Service program for them. Instead of going into the military, they built roads, worked in mental hospitals, became smoke jumpers, and did other public service jobs. Later, during the Korean and

Good Sense from the Good Folks of Iowa

Vietnam wars, a classification of 1-W gave COs opportunity again to work in public service.

Some people confuse us with the Amish. The Amish and Mennonites are alike when it comes to beliefs about God, but the Amish believe in being separate from the "world" while Mennonites live a more contemporary lifestyle. No doubt you have seen the distinctively dressed Amish driving around Kalona in horse-and-buggies.

Both Amish and Mennonites express their beliefs by working with the Mennonite Central Committee in many parts of the world. Remember I told you I taught in Newfoundland? That was in voluntary service with the Mennonite Central Committee. Both groups also work with the Mennonite Disaster Service, volunteering to serve in areas beset by fire, flood, and other disasters.

There you have it—a small picture of a small religious group mightily important to Iowa. I hope you will respond with your ideas of what makes a good life in Iowa.

Always, your "old" teacher,

Lois Gugel

Cary J. Hahn

Cary J. Hahn has been CBS 2 KGAN-TV's "Iowa Traveler" feature reporter in Cedar Rapids since 1983. In 2006, The Iowa Broadcast News Association (IBNA) honored the eastern Iowa broadcast veteran with their prestigious Jack Shelley Award. The award is the IBNA's highest honor and is named after the former WHO news director and professor emeritus of journalism at Iowa State University.

Dear Young Iowan:

As the Iowa Traveler, I've been around—around the state and halfway around the world as a Vietnam War sailor.

But it may surprise you to know I'm not a native Iowan. I came to Iowa in 1979, having grown up in Missouri. I've now lived longer in Iowa than in my native state. Both are great places, and both have produced great people, not to mention lasting friends.

My favorite president was from Missouri: Harry S Truman. He had one daughter, Margaret, to whom he wrote many letters. In one he said, "Your dad will never be reckoned with the great. But you can be sure he did his level best and gave all he had to his country. There is an epitaph in Boot Hill Cemetery in Tombstone, Arizona, which reads, 'Here lies Jack Williams; he done his damnedest.' What more can a person do?"

Harry S Truman was an "accidental president," inheriting the job when President Franklin D. Roosevelt died and after Mr. Truman had served only eighty-two days as vice president.

But Harry's experience as a Missouri farmer, World War I Army captain, small business owner, county judge, and U.S. Senator all counted when he became our nation's chief executive. On his desk, a sign read: "The Buck Stops Here." He took responsibility and dedicated himself to public service.

More than a half century has passed since President Truman left office. Historians have looked at his record and many put him at the top of the list of great Presidents. It appears he did his damnedest.

The nation's only Iowa-born president is Herbert Hoover. Sadly, many people think of him only as the president who was in office when the Great Depression began. However, take a visit to the Hoover Presidential Library and Museum in his hometown of West Branch, Iowa and you will discover he was a great humanitarian in charge of feeding millions of starving people after both World Wars.

Truman was a Democrat, Hoover a Republican. That did not stop them from being friends. It was Truman, after all, who asked Hoover to help with the European recovery after World War II. Writing to Truman in 1962, the fellow former president told Truman, "Yours has been a friendship which has reached deeper into my life than you know.

"My country owes me nothing. It gave me, as it gives every boy and girl, a chance. It gave me schooling, independence of action, opportunity for service and honor. In no other land could a boy from a country village, without inheritance or influential friends, look forward with unbounded hope."

Hoover said that, but Truman might just as well have said it.

The point is this: Make lasting friends and be proud to call yourself an Iowan. Go out and do your ... well, you know.

Sincerely,

Cary J. Hahn

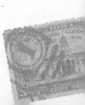

Morgan Halgren

Morgan Halgren was raised in Parkville, Missouri, where her parents owned and operated a summer theater on the acreage where they lived. In college Halgren studied Spanish, French, and German and, after a brief stint as a flight attendant for TWA, she went to graduate school at Indiana University.

In 1971 she and her husband, Dr. Carl Halgren, moved to Iowa. Since that time she has made a career as a freelance media talent doing radio and television commercials, narrations, public speaking, training and industrial films, and on-hold messages for businesses around the country. Recently retired from twenty-seven years as a host of a weekly magazine show on Iowa Public Television, Living in Iowa, *she continues in her role as the lead singer for a Latin jazz group known as Sabrosa. Both her daughters live in Europe.*

Dear Young Iowan:

I could tell by the tone of your voice that you were happy, and when we hung up the phone, I said to your dad, "She's going to stay in Europe." That was over a decade ago, and since that time you have married a Dutchman, earned dual citizenship, worked all over Europe as a business consultant, given birth to a beautiful little boy, and blessed us with the promise of another child to arrive, appropriately, around Thanksgiving. You have made your life there, and it suits you well.

It took me several years to accept this decision and understand it. I remember when your dad had a sabbatical from his teaching and he decided to do research in Holland for a semester so that we could be near you. You were studying at Leiden University and living in a wonderful, old student house that had been built around 1740. You found us a nice apartment in the same town, and went to great trouble to furnish it for us.

I remember one night I left your student house and began walking slowly to our apartment. It was a turning point for me. Bricks in careful patterns drew me down alleys where small homes hid like sweet surprises. Windows with nothing to hide caught my eye and invited me to imagine their owners. I pictured the typical tall Dutch man or woman with their quiet reserve, their ease of navigating on a bike or ice skates. Having met your friends, I knew that the Dutch relish the fine art of conversation fueled by dark coffee and pastries coaxed from a nearby oven. I understood your attraction to their ability to express their true opinions on any topic, and their respect when you expressed an opposing view. And then I wondered if your ears, like theirs, were now accustomed to the sounds of seagulls, street organs, market days and the bells of ancient churches.

As I walked on, I passed the famous street where a group of pilgrims who came to America lived before they bravely crossed the ocean, and I could feel history in my feet. It was then I understood that a part of me had taken root in Leiden, taken root behind a door that had opened against two and a half centuries of time. My brave pilgrim daughter was that part of me. Her heart had crossed an ocean, and her voice had found a cadence of its own.

You tell me that people there comment on your friendliness, your great work ethic, and your enthusiasm. Your Dutch friends tell me they have never had a friend like you—so loyal, such a good listener, so thoughtful. So now, dear daughter, I think of you as our courageous ambassador from Iowa who, by virtue of her personality, shows the old world every day that a small state in the new world is a place worth knowing about.

Love always,

Mom

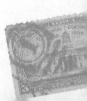

David Hamilton

A native Missourian and a longtime resident of Iowa City, David Hamilton teaches at the University of Iowa, where he edits The Iowa Review. *The son of a farmer-engineer-archaeologist-historian, Hamilton extends his family's long commitment to natural and regional history in his experimental memoir* Deep River: A Memoir of a Missouri Farm. *His most recent book is* Ossabaw, *a book of poems from Salt Publications in Cambridge, England.*

Dear Young Iowan:

Is it possible that you still write letters?

My family treasures several stashes from our past, each of which came from one of us spending a year, or a few, in Russia, Colombia, Gabon, or Prague. Each bundle proves the writer found a quiet place and the uninterrupted moment needed for introspection—an intimacy born of pen and paper. An intimacy, so far as I know, peculiar to letters. Another collection came from Iowa in the 1920s, when my father wrote to his farm parents in what seemed then a distant, neighboring state.

The letters from the Russian-Polish frontier, which are from about the same time, became the first draft of a book.

Suppose you had gone with me this summer to France, as a group of our students did. *Bonjour,* people say to us on the street, and they say it as if they mean it. *Bonjour,* a man says broadly as he enters a café, speaking to those being served as well as to those serving. There are further exchanges with men behind the counter, even a handshake over the shoulders of customers standing nearer to it. Nor does our customer leave without bidding *adieu.* There is no tight little silent smile of greeting—almost a grimace—or slipping away with barely a nod.

On our trip we notice other things as well: toilets that differentiate a larger from a smaller flush and so use less water; washing machines that also conserve water but get clothes just as clean; an absence of parking meters in favor of small, automatic kiosks, one or two per block, from which you acquire tickets; traffic circles allowing for the convenience of rolling, right hand turns; toll roads on which the hard-working truckers stay in the right lane, at a lower speed, governed rather than governing.

Together we admire the wide boulevards and many parks of Paris and, out in the country, sycamores—"plane trees"—lining the road. Farm kids at heart, we comment on the dry-stone walls snaking up the sides of mountains, defining ancient gardens and fields. Hikers, sometimes boisterous, sometimes winded, startle us. A kestrel, slightly larger than ours back home in the States, hovers above high meadows. Magenta foxglove grows as lush in the wild as hybrids in our Iowa gardens. A blackbird sings, really sings, as the old rhyme suggests. His voice is melodic.

Let me imagine you then staying on in France for some time after our summer program ends. There, on your own, and experiencing some loneliness no doubt, you may seek out that quiet, inner place that a letter defines and into which we invite only our best friends. You will have plenty to write about since differences abound, and you will have honed your ability to notice them. Writing of all that, and more, your letters may begin to say *come join me* in so many words, as the quiet scratch of the pen on paper becomes, perhaps, a lover's whisper.

Perhaps, too, your writing will slow and you will pay more attention to your hand, something you cared less about when you were in school. You may even find yourself growing envious of your grandparents' penmanship, the product of a little school a long time ago. You will probably stifle that nostalgia, but may it flicker for you like the rumor of an all-but-forgotten folklore.

By now you will have discovered, too, the pleasure of notebooks in textures different from those you could have purchased at home, some of which prove irresistible. You just have to buy them. You will purchase several and plan each for a different project and then, if you are like me, you'll not stick to your plan.

Meanwhile, your correspondence unfurls, as leaves on a tree. On the privacy of handwritten pages, you will have plumbed your mind in a way face-to-face conversations, much less electronic ones with all their quick interruptions, do not allow. Perhaps you will have put yourself across so well that your correspondent will be joining you soon, wherever you are, and that is cause to celebrate! If not, your pages may at least have gathered like the leaves of a book, which will be some compensation—if books prove to be something your generation still writes.

Sincerely yours,

David Hamilton

Neil E. Harl

Born on a rented farm in southern Iowa, Neil E. Harl attended a one-room country school for eight years, graduated from Seymour High School in 1951, and enrolled at Iowa State College. After two years of active duty with the U.S. Army as an artillery officer and a year as a farm magazine writer, he earned a law degree at the University of Iowa and a PhD in economics from Iowa State.

Since joining the faculty at Iowa State University over forty years ago, the prolific Harl has authored twenty-eight books and over nine hundred articles in farm and financial publications. These publications, in addition to his distinguished record of teaching some nine thousand ISU students over the years, earned Harl the Charles F. Curtiss Distinguished Professor in Agriculture in 1976. Supremely versatile, he has been president of the American Agricultural Economics Association and the first president of the American Agricultural Law Association in addition to serving on six federal commissions.

Dear Young Iowan:

My advice for you is to be alert to opportunities to make yourself a better person, a person who is better equipped to serve the human family. Rewards will surely come to you as you develop yourself for the life ahead. Watch for those key decisions that have the potential to shape your life. Sometimes those decisions are not posed to you with flags flying and with a dramatic drumroll announcing that a highly important decision lay just ahead.

A challenge can make all the difference, and I aim to challenge you, too. Dad's challenge to me when I started at a one-room country school, the Hays School, in the autumn of 1939, was that if I worked hard in the primary grade (there was no kindergarten then; it was called "primary") and passed both primary and first grade in my first year in school, he would give me an ewe lamb. I viewed that as a big reward, something worth being competitive for. And it made an indelible impression on me.

Without a doubt the most critical decision in my life was the decision to go to college at Iowa State. My parents were disappointed with the decision and made that clear to me at various times. Perhaps I should explain why I believe the decision to go to college was so important. While it is certainly possible to grow and develop intellectually and socially in other settings, college provides an intensive, focused period for personal development. It is more than developing the abilities to write, to speak, and to think, important as those are to one's development. It also involves the ability to relate to others as young adults, to learn how to build and sustain relationships, and to function in a world of independence.

When I graduated from high school in 1951, the world was a much different place than it is today. Globalization, international trade, and "outsourcing" have combined to send a clear message to high school graduates of the twenty-first century in the United States. If you want to spend a lifetime competing for employment with individuals with limited education, the choice is a relatively easy one. But if you want a better, more satisfying life, every year of additional education beyond high school is a good investment. Every degree, every level upward reduces the number in the world with whom you will be competing. If you choose a career path wisely, you are likely to be rewarded. But remember, there is no assurance of an easy life no matter how many degrees you attain.

And life hasn't always been easy for me, nor have I always won. I was terribly disappointed that I was turned down as the farm tenant on the Cover Farm, which we later purchased from the Cover family in 2002. The refusal came after I had completed college and two years of military service and felt otherwise worthy.

Hopes for a career in farming dashed, I began pursuing what had earlier appeared to be a good job opportunity—the executive training program at General Mills in Minneapolis. I drove as far as Des Moines and stopped to call my cousin, David Bryant, who was working as a field editor at *Wallaces Farmer*. He told me that he was leaving the position and his job had not been filled. I called the editor, Richard Albrecht, and was hired on the spot. So instead of accepting employment with General Mills in Minneapolis, I signed on as a writer in Des Moines. The second most important move of my life was the decision to go back to school—to law school and to graduate school. I happened to be at the University of Iowa at just the right time, early June of 1958, interviewing Professor John C. O'Byrne for three stories I was working on. He gave me almost a half day of his time. And then he posed a surprising question: was I interested in going back to school for a law degree and a PhD in economics? He explained that he and John Timmons of Iowa State College had just reached an agreement on sponsoring someone to get both degrees. I was momentarily stunned. I had been thinking about graduate school but it seemed like a remote dream. Now an opportunity was opening up right before my eyes. When I walked out of Professor O'Byrne's office late that afternoon, I knew that my life had forever been changed. The scary part of that decision was the happenstance involved, and I relate it to you now because it suggests something about serendipity and the good fortune of staying light on your feet.

Above all, young Iowan, do your level best in everything you do, whether it is in academics, athletics, business, a profession, or in a relationship with the love of your life. Our span of time on this earth is relatively short. Make the most of it.

With my love and best wishes,

Neil Harl

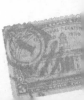

Phyllis Harris

Phyllis Harris, who returned to Ames in 2003, writes that she always considered herself an Iowan despite having lived more than twice as many years in Illinois as in her native Iowa. Born and raised in Ames, she attended what was then Iowa State College, though interests in the liberal arts led her to the University of Minnesota, where she ultimately received her undergraduate degree.

A kindergarten teacher, she earned a Master's from the University of Illinois and, more recently, a Master of Fine Arts in writing from the low-residency program at Vermont College. Her essays have appeared in the Chicago Tribune; *fiction in* Ranger Rick; *and poems in* Lyrical Iowa. *Her book titles include* Stories From Where We Live: Great Lakes Edition *from Milkweed Press and* Celebrating Family History *from Southern California Genealogical Society. Harris, feeling more comfortable with poetry, writes her letter to a young Iowan as a prose-poem.*

Dear Young Iowan:

As a born and bred Iowan myself,
One who has lived all her married life in a neighboring industrial state,
One who, as a widow returning to Iowa, left her children
And grandchildren in that neighboring state,
I have a vision and a secret to share with you.

The vision first:
Just as Americans went westward ho in the nineteenth and twentieth
        centuries,
Just as Californians more recently invaded Washington and Oregon,
Just as the eastern seaboard suffers from city snarl and highway glut,
Iowa beckons with less, yes *less:*
Less population density,
Less crowded scenic highways,
But *more* work ethic that continues to shine.

While I lived my fifty years in another state,
Strangers moved into Iowa and laid claim to all

My grandfather and father held dear before me.
And why not? Once these strangers relocated
They recognized Iowa's comfort zone.

Even with children living in other states
These newcomers chose to remain in Iowa,
Knowing that the quality of life elsewhere
Is one others in retirement
Yearn to flee.

I read stories in the *Chicago Tribune* about successful
Entrepreneurs, scientists, engineers, chemists, writers, to name but
    a few
Who, the stories go, were born in Iowa
And educated in one of Iowa's universities.
Every time the word "wholesome" came to mind.

It's been said (by me) that in some ways Vermont,
About which much is written, romanticized, and sung, is
A more sophisticated version of Iowa. It has the landscape,
The good people, the work ethic, and many new residents
Fleeing New York City.
Just as Vermont is considered a haven for the East
Iowa emerges as the refuge of the future.

We know what happens to procrastinators.
Sometimes the human body takes exception to our plans
Regarding length of life.
Sometimes we fail to listen to that still small voice within
That cheers what is known and loved too well to gain notice
Until we leave.

It has been said that mentally most of us continue to live
And relive our childhood years, so influential are they
Despite later adult lifestyles in rarefied places.

And now for the secret:
I was careful to bring my children to Iowa from that neighboring state
Every summer of their formative years.
I saw to it that
My out-of-state children were fully indoctrinated
With Iowa sweet corn, raspberries, the dairy barn, summer evenings,
Grant Wood, Herbert Hoover, Christian Petersen, Clear Lake, the
    neighbors
And now
A daughter has infected
My son-in-law.
He simply can't be cured
Until he locates
In Iowa.

Phil Hey

Phil Hey has been teaching and gardening in Sioux City since 1969, before which he received his Master of Fine Arts degree from the University of Iowa in 1966. He was raised in Illinois but considers himself a convert to Iowa. He is author of the book How It Seems to Me.

Dear Young Iowan:

I've just come in from working on my garden—mulching and watering tomatoes and peppers, and once again figuring out how to keep the weeds away—and it seems like a fine time to write you. So what's worth saying after living in Iowa these past thirty-seven years?

Here's a good beginning: *love the people.* Yeah, I know, you think of all the people you dislike, their bad tastes and prejudices, perhaps most of all their sense of ownership—what Iowan Meredith Willson in *The Music Man* called "Iowa stubborn."

And so you imagine getting away from them, somehow leaving them behind forever, and one way or another it's going to happen. People leave Iowa all the time, moving to places like California (which is most of what you see on TV), and what do they do there? They form Iowa clubs! Who could have guessed? So you could move, too.

But what I'm really thinking about here is the wonderful people you might never get to know, whether you move away or stay in Iowa and they pass on before you come to know them well enough. What Iowans as people are known for isn't their slickness—leave that to Californians—or their snobbery or their money. (Would you want to have Donald Trump as a neighbor?)

Of the words I've tried to fit to the Iowans I know, two keep sounding right: Iowans are kind and wise. For kindness, you can read stories in the *Des Moines Register* almost every day about how an Iowan helped out someone from somewhere else (yes, a complete stranger) without expecting money or recognition. And along almost every local road or street you'll have people wave to you, even if you don't wave first. It just seems right, doesn't it?

About wisdom, it's hard to define, but you might know it well when you see it. Yes, historically, Iowans have been smart, well-educated, and thoughtful citizens about public issues, but that's not all of wisdom. Part of what I associate with wisdom is deliberateness, taking time to think over a problem or a decision, and another part is humaneness—what would be right for the people or the land? Again, you won't see much of it on TV, or see it in ads about how some new gadget will suddenly change your life; leave that to people who want to live on the surface of things. Iowa may be a good place for wisdom because we understand, literally, about putting down roots, about how the finest speechifying in the world won't make anything grow better, and the sun comes up only one day at a time. You know how that goes; you live here, too.

So, if you do move somewhere, you won't have to work too hard to remember that Iowa and its people made you much of what you are. And if you stay in Iowa, let yourself be known for the land and people you love. You couldn't do better.

Fondly,

Phil Hey

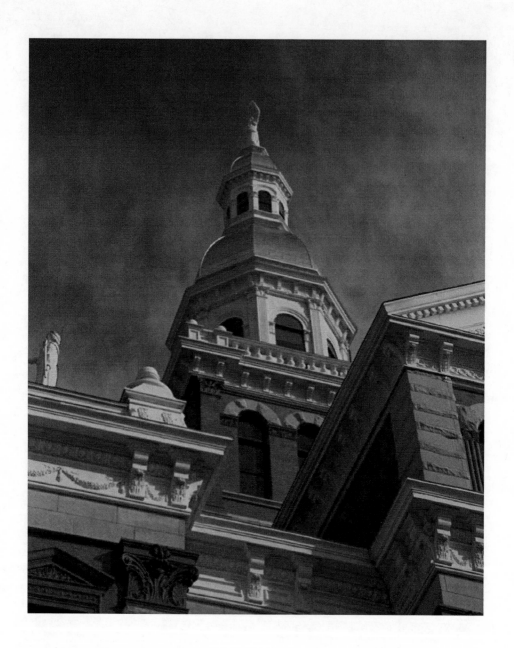

Photographs © Michael Harker

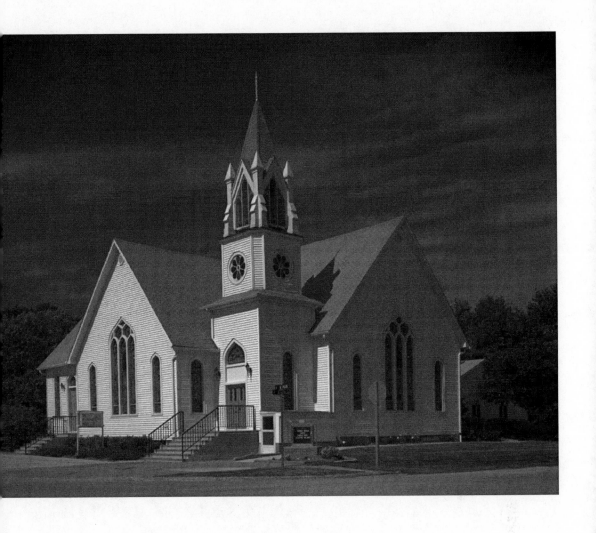

Jim Heynen

Born on a farm in northwest Iowa in one of the last areas of the state to get electricity, Jim Heynen also attended one of the last one-room schoolhouses. He attended Hull Western Christian High, then two years at Dordt College in Sioux Center before going on to receive his BA at Calvin College in Grand Rapids, Michigan. Heynen then returned to his native state and the University of Iowa for an MA in English Renaissance literature before earning his MFA at the University of Oregon.

Jim Heynen is best known for his short-short stories about farm boys. He has published widely as a writer of poems, novels, nonfiction, and short fiction. His stories about "the boys" have been featured often on National Public Radio's All Things Considered, *and the most recent collection of these stories,* The Boys' House, *was named Editors' Choice for Best Books 2001 by the* Bloomsbury Review, Newsday, *and* Booklist. *Heynen is writer-in-residence at St. Olaf College in Northfield, Minnesota, in between frequent trips back to his home state of Iowa.*

Dear Young Iowan:

My father, your great-grandfather, liked to think that you were like David in the Bible. You were your great-grandfather's favorite, and he thought you were one who would live up to a name that carries so much meaning: *David*, Beloved. You were expected to be a person of valor, a natural leader, and someone whose language would follow the tradition of the David who wrote the Psalms. Like David, you are the youngest, learning from your older siblings while finding your own particular way of being in the world.

David, I trust the future to you, I really do. When I was a boy on the farm—right across the road from where you live now—we were not concerned about the damage we might be doing with DDT, 2-4D, and a host of other pesticides and herbicides. We were out to conquer the land and animals. Many years later, when I watched you as a boy of eight coaxing your pet chicken to come to your call, I knew your great-grandfather was right about you: you were different. I knew your way in the world would be extraordinary and special. A pet chicken? Good grief! I hated chickens. Everybody hated chickens. We considered chickens the epitome of brainlessness among animals—and yet I saw you do something that I never in my life saw anyone do before: you called to a chicken and it came running! A chicken! That fat waddling black chicken came running to you like an admiring and intelligent trained dog. It was a little bit spooky to see a stupid chicken actually come to the call of a boy. A little bit spooky, but also quite amazing. I had the feeling that if you had held out your hand to that chicken it would have laid a golden egg in it.

This is more a letter of apology than a letter of advice. Like other farm boys before you, you have seen the births and deaths of animals. Like me, you learned the facts of life early and knew both the beauty of animals coming into the world and the sadness of seeing them sent off to market or dying from diseases and accidents. But I apologize for how many wild creatures we eliminated before you got here. I'm sorry that in our rage for more efficient production we did away with most of the pheasants, all of the Hungarian partridge, all of the badgers, most of the skunks, all of the jack rabbits, all of the red-headed woodpeckers, all of the brown thrashers, all of the chickenhawks, all of the pocket gophers, all of the mud turtles, all of the weasels—even all of the rats. It's not as if rats were fun, but I wish you could at least have seen them scurrying out of the corncribs after a rainstorm to sip water from the puddles. I'm sorry we d-Conned every last one of them out of existence. I think you would have found the rats interesting, and you probably would have tamed a few and kept them as pets.

You'll soon be hit by the madness of adolescence—the call to compete in sports, the call of the video games, the call to break the strict rules of our conservative community. I want to tell you that I am not worried about you. You know how to call the most vulnerable (and, yes, stupid) of the world to you. This is not a skill, it is a gift. I might warn you to preserve what is left of the landscape and its creatures, but I know I don't have to preach to you. All I would tell you is to honor your gift. Call the world to you, and I believe it will be as good to you as you clearly are inclined to be toward it.

With respect and love,

Your Uncle Jim

Vicky Hinsenbrock

Vicky Hinsenbrock graduated from Iowa State University with a degree in animal science and currently works for the United States Department of Agriculture. These twin interests—agriculture and animal science—also keep her busy at home on a small acreage outside Decorah, where she and her husband keep dogs, cats, horses, and cattle. A true devotee of Iowa as well as a native, she has lived in the state all but one year of her life. Hinsenbrock is perhaps best known for co-authoring, with Ruth Hein, the book, Ghostly Tales of Iowa, *though she also publishes magazine articles. She happily reports she does not share her 1883 Victorian home with ghosts, at least none that she knows of.*

Dear Young Iowan:

Even native Iowans do not think of Iowa as having the classic "haunted houses" or ghostly visitors. But we do.

Writer Ruth Hein and I spent many hours researching stories and talking to ordinary Iowans about just that—ghosts and ghostly tales. Our research put us in touch with a variety of ages, occupations, and ethnic backgrounds. We talked with young people, old people, men, women, and even small children—all Iowans. What they had in common was their belief that something—inexplicable as it might be—had happened to them, their relatives, their neighbors. They were, as we Iowans are, a bit reserved, especially about such topics as ghosts and haunted houses.

But talk they did.

They called us, wrote us letters, faxed us, set up interviews. Iowans had stories about unexplained noises—footsteps, ghostly dogs, voices whispered in the night—and stories about haunted homes and shadowy visitors. Some stories were one hundred years old and some happened just recently. Some happened at colleges, some at seemingly ordinary homes. The one thing that stood out, and still stands out, was an Iowans' need to share: to tell someone else what had happened or was happening, to carry on important oral stories.

What stories do you have to share, young Iowan, and how do we, you and I, reconcile these supernatural stories with the traditional view of Iowans as upright, solid, decent, hard-working people who perhaps lack a little in imagination? By that logic, are those Iowans prone to ghostly witness gifted with more imagination than the rest of us?

Probably not.

Such stories came from all over the state—from the old German river town of Guttenberg, to Des Moines, to Davenport, another river town, to Okoboji in northwest Iowa. During our book promotion visits throughout the state, not once did we leave without hearing more stories from our eager audiences. Iowans believed these supernatural stories, and we believed in these Iowans.

Perhaps what we need to do here is challenge traditional disbelief. Are we hard-working and honest people?—you bet we are. But we are also, judging by my experience, a people who can believe in the inexplicable.

I have always been proud to be an Iowan, and I hope, young Iowan, you will be, too. And I hope we will always have room in our hearts for the mysterious.

Sincerely,

Vicky

Good Sense from the Good Folks of Iowa

Bruce and Jeanette Hopkins

Bruce Hopkins is a writer, educator, and environmentalist who served as chief administrator of Western Hills Area Education Agency in Sioux City before his recent retirement. Bruce has taught at every level of education: as a teacher of criminology and black studies in Nebraska and New York, as a staff member at Iowa State University in Ames, and as a visiting professor at Colorado College and the University of Louisiana. He exhibited as part of an interactive art exhibit at the University of Dubuque with Francisco Licarrdi; in the Hudson River Valley arts exhibit in the Catskill Mountains, and the Lake Arts Center in the Adirondack Mountains of New York.

Jeanette Hopkins has been a middle and elementary educator for over twenty years. She is currently an adjunct professor at Morningside College in Sioux City. Jeanette is a member of the advisory board for the Iowa Writing Project, a nonprofit organization designed to encourage a natural approach to writing in the classroom. Bruce and Jeanette both facilitate "A Sense of Place" writing workshops throughout the Midwest and present annually at the Loess Hills Prairie Seminar in northwest Iowa.

Dear Young Iowan:

> We never speak, for example, of an environment we have known;
> it is always places we have known … and recall. We are homesick
> for places; it is the sounds and smells and sights of places which
> haunt us and against which we often measure our present.
> —Alan Gussow

When I was preparing to leave for college, my high school science teacher shared a small piece of wisdom. He told me that I would never really leave the Sand Hills of Nebraska as there would come a time, later in life, when they would call me "home." Though I didn't return to live in the Sand Hills of my youth, I did find "home" in the Loess Hills of Iowa.

As we have visited with Iowans these past few months, we've found that each person has indicated a strong need to find notions of place, stories, and experiences that provide some meaning. In *Having Everything Right*, writer Kim Stafford shares how, for the Kwakiutl People of the Northwest coast, a name *was* a story. For example, a patch of ocean became "Where Salmon Gather"; each name represented the situation or experience of the tribal people. Stafford laments our lack of understanding in knowing place, and examines the potential of joining signifying stories and histories with present practices of naming place and experience.

For you, as a young Iowan, it really doesn't matter where your feet land, but what matters tremendously is your ability to know and understand where you have landed.

In 1977, a young educator-naturalist, Carolyn Benne, organized the first Loess Hills Prairie Seminar in northwest Iowa. This seminar has come to be a living memorial to Carolyn's dreams that all children and adults experience the idea of a "total village," wherein schools and communities come together to share and learn of the natural world—the prairie of northwest Iowa—and how to protect it. We hope you will experience this place in Iowa as one young child did a few years ago when, as she stood overlooking the Big Sioux River and Red Tail Ridge in northwest Iowa, she could see the bluestem grass, prairie coneflowers, and hear the whispers of native legends. Emily knew the stories of how the native storyteller from the past could be heard even today if one listened carefully to the grasses. She remembers this day of discovery as the best in her life.

The process of *being* an Iowan is an active one where the seeker, the student-citizen—you—come to recognize the nature of growing in knowledge and insight, growing *in place*. Too often we Iowans look around us to find that our neighbors have an enhanced sense of what makes their state unique. The Black Hills of South Dakota, the lakes of Minnesota, the Ozarks of Missouri, and the Sand Hills of Nebraska are only aspects of each place. As you take up the art of representing place—whether in a poem, a painting, or a natural history—refrain from replicating the ideal of other regions. Embrace this place we call home. If you come to northwest Iowa and you feel the positive spirit in the hills, let us know. We'll invite you to hear more stories, and to name these new experiences in a very special way.

Brion Hurley

Brion Hurley grew up in Iowa City, where he attended Helen Lemme Elementary, Southeast Junior High School, City High School, and the University of Iowa for a BA in statistics and an MA in quality management. The epitome of an Iowa student-athlete, Hurley walked-on to the University of Iowa's football team in 1992, earning a full scholarship one year later. After concluding a successful athletic and academic career at Iowa in 1996, Hurley was invited to attend the New York Giants National Football League training camp in 1997 and 1999 and, in between, played for the Iowa Barnstormers in the Arena Football League. Hurley formally concluded his football career in 2001 after two straight championship seasons with the Arena 2 Football League's Quad City Steamwheelers. Now a successful statistician, Brion Hurley works for Rockwell Collins, most recently at their Melbourne, Florida facility.

Dear Young Iowan:

Deciding which college to attend is probably the biggest decision you will make in your young life. It is never an easy decision, especially when it might mean traveling hundreds or thousands of miles away from home.

The lure of moving to a new town or city, where no one knows who you are, to attend a "big name" program always entices. Take it from me; it seems like you have really "made it" when schools from all over the country—the very schools that once seemed unattainable to you—come calling.

I'm asking that you consider the strength of Iowa colleges one more time. Although Iowa does not offer professional sports teams, huge metropolitan cities, and sunshine year round, what it does offer overshadows all of those things.

Iowans work hard. Most Iowans learned that work ethic from working on the farm, and others learned it from their friends, teachers, coaches, or parents—mentors who had to model that very same work ethic in order to stay competitive in their jobs. However, the work ethic that you grew up with and have come to expect of others does not always exist everywhere else. You will be disappointed that others, whom you rely on for academic or athletic success, do not always share those some traits. Even so, those with a strong work ethic will come through for you, whether it's to help you complete a major project in class or to make that crucial free throw to win the game.

Iowans are well-educated. Without the distractions of big city living and the need to "keep up with the Joneses," Iowans can afford to focus on the important things, such as creating the very best schools for their children. The education you have received in Iowa, then, is one of the best in the nation. There are high expectations of you as a student, and graduating high school is the first step in achieving those expectations.

Achieving a degree from an Iowa college or university is a great honor and will serve you well when you look for a job in the future. You could also get a degree from another reputable school, but it will be very expensive. Especially if you have to pay out-of-state tuition, your investment may be slow to pay off.

The freedom of being away from home means that you can do what you want, and you won't be held immediately accountable for your actions. If you slack off and don't succeed as an athlete, not many people from home will find out. If you get marginal grades, only your family will probably know.

However, when you stay in Iowa, you will be expected to succeed. When you are not succeeding, people will ask why, but also will be willing to help, if needed. This may be tough to handle when things aren't going well, but when you do start to succeed, you will hear praise from everyone, even those whom you have never met before.

My athletic experience at the University of Iowa will be remembered favorably by most Iowans even though it was not always an easy road. I cannot help but think, for example, of the numerous games where I felt responsible for a Hawkeye loss. In a nutshell, the ups and downs of my career were as follows:

+ Named first-team punter prior to 1993 season
+ Lost job after third game
+ Took over kickoff duties
+ Took over as placekicker for final game of the year and the 1993
  Alamo Bowl that followed; made my first field goal in 37-3 loss

- Earned a full-ride football scholarship
- Lost placekicking job during spring practice
- Gained placekicking job back midway through the 1994 season
- Had three point-after attempts blocked in first game as placekicker in 1994 in loss to Oregon
- Missed late field goal attempt (too low) against Michigan, ending comeback
- Kicked two field goals against Michigan State in 19-14 victory
- Completed 1994 season with fourteen point-after attempts in last two games
- Missed point-after attempt in first game of 1995 season, and missed short field goal against rival Iowa State in next game; lost job permanently after the game
- Brought in for long field goals in game versus Michigan State; made 51-yarder
- Hit 50-yard field goal versus Wisconsin
- Earned Sun Bowl Special Teams MVP for three long field goals in win over Washington
- Connected on 54-yard field goal in 1996 against rival Iowa State (sweet revenge)
- Kicked 51-yard field goal versus Michigan State to help fuel comeback win
- Booted 50-yard field goal against Minnesota

I share my athletic "resumé" for two reasons. First, everyone must deal with disappointments in order to reach their goals. Second, each of these setbacks made me stronger, and the support of my family, teammates, coaches, friends, and fans allowed me to overcome. They were able to forgive some of my errors, because, as an Iowan, they knew I was trying hard. I was forgiven, but also expected to bounce back and perform. I couldn't disappear after a few bad games because people were able to follow my performance very closely. They were holding me accountable.

In the end, I believe that I wouldn't have had the success I did had I attended a college outside of Iowa. There are many other advantages of staying in Iowa for your higher education, but for me they boil down to education, work ethic, and accountability.

Sincerely,

Brion Hurley

Patrick Irelan

Birmingham, the Iowa town where Patrick Irelan was conceived, and Fairfield, the Iowa town where he was born, seem in retrospect, according to Irelan, fated for these purposes. Pete and Gerata Hunter Irelan chose each other, but the mighty Chicago, Burlington & Quincy Railroad—"Everywhere West"—chose where his parents would work, and, therefore, where they would be fruitful and multiply. Irelan attended a one-room country school in Davis County, worked on the family's eighty-acre farm, and graduated from the same high school as his parents and his sister, Jane. After graduation, he would go on to earn a BA and MA from the University of Iowa and raise two daughters, Clare and Emily. Ultimately, Irelan would work for his alma mater at the University of Iowa's Division of Continuing Education until his retirement in 2004.

Irelan's publications include many short stories and essays; a family memoir, Central Standard: A Time, a Place, a Family; *and a personal memoir,* A Firefly in the Night. *He is presently working on a collection of short stories.*

Dear Young Iowan:

You have a good history teacher. She is entirely correct in saying that a network of passenger trains and streetcars once provided transportation for every part of Iowa. I think this system and its ultimate destruction will make a fine subject for your class project. And since Ms. Noland urged you to seek the help of your grandparents, I'll be happy to pass along any memories I can.

I recall the last years of this passenger system and rode on every train or streetcar that still existed near the little farm where I grew up. As I've told you many times, your great-grandfather Pete worked for two of the largest railroads west of the Mississippi, and he often let me go with him to the depots where he worked for the Rock Island Railroad in Iowa towns like Centerville, Seymour, and Allerton. These hours spent with my father still give me the fondest memories of my childhood.

Your great-grandfather held strong opinions about the decline of passenger-train service, and he had the evidence to back up his opinions. I'll give you one example: Certain auto, oil, tire, and related companies used every means they could to replace trains and streetcars with cars and buses. In 1949, in a trial that hardly anyone remembers, a federal jury in Chicago found General Motors, Standard Oil of California, Phillips Petroleum, Firestone Tire, Mack Manufacturing, and other corporations guilty of buying streetcar systems, replacing them with bus systems, and selling them to companies that agreed to buy buses, fuel, and tires from only the corporations involved in this conspiracy. These actions violated the Sherman Antitrust Act of 1890.

I have a collection of articles about events like these, and I'll copy them for you. But to make your presentation really succeed, you'll need to go beyond laws, trials, and criminal conspiracies. You need to give your teacher and the other students a sense of what we've lost. Fortunately, we still have Amtrak. Let your grandpa drive over and pick you up next Saturday. We'll go to Mount Pleasant, to the same depot where your great-grandfather worked in the 1940s. We'll get there thirty minutes early and watch the crowd gather. Passengers are often nervous about when the train will arrive. Try to sense their emotions. Listen to them talk to each other. Listen to the way the depot agent reassures them. You'll hear the same words I heard when I was a boy.

Then we'll go out onto the depot platform to wait for the eastbound California Zephyr. We're sure to see at least one coal train while we're waiting, and it may be going faster than the Burlington Northern Santa Fe railroad really wants it to go. Some engineers never grow up. They remain boys until they retire, and they love the speed and muscle of those four big freight locomotives.

Then, in the distance, we'll see the three lights of the first Genesis locomotive. Two of these locomotives pull train No. 6 all the way from the San Francisco Bay to Chicago. We'll hear two short bursts and one long blast of the whistle for each grade crossing. As the train comes closer, listen to the warning bells and watch the red lights flashing as the gates go down at the street just west of the depot.

Watch for the conductor at an open door, talking by hand-held radio to the engineer. Conductors still used hand or lantern signals when I was your age. Watch how gently the train comes to a stop, and how quickly the conductor steps down and sets the Pullman stool on the platform. See the other crew members step down at other doors. Watch how calmly the conductor greets the passengers. This is an act. The conductor isn't really calm. Passenger-train conductors cannot stand the sight of a motionless train.

Take all this in. Never forget it for the rest of your life. Leave your camera and tape recorder at home. Put it into words. Nothing is more powerful than words written and rewritten until they are perfect. And you have that power because you were born with it.

You'll describe that scene perfectly, because I already have two round-trip tickets for Chicago, and you can start writing as soon as we find our seats, or you can wait until later because you may want to see every vista as train No. 6 accelerates away from the depot, bound for the train shed at Union Station, 2438 miles from the San Francisco Bay.

Pack your bags. I'm getting nervous. The train leaves in only seven days.

Love,

Grandpa

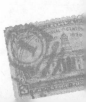

Jan Jensen

Associate head coach of the University of Iowa women's basketball team and Iowa Girls High School Basketball Hall-of-Famer Jan Jensen serves as the recruiting coordinator for the Hawkeyes and also works with the post players, efforts which have helped guide Iowa to six straight postseason appearances and a Big Ten Tournament championship in 2001.

In her senior year at Drake University, Jensen led the nation in scoring with 29.6 points per game, collecting honors as a Kodak Honorable Mention All-American, a GTE Academic All-America Player of the Year, and a Sports Illustrated *National Player of the Week. Jensen is one of only two Drake players to have her number retired in Drake's Knapp Center. After college, Jensen played professionally in the European Professional Basketball League for BTV-Wuppertal in Germany. Jensen's parents, Dale and Yvonne, reside in Kimballton along with her brother, Doug, and niece Ashley. Her older sister, Melodi Jenkins, lives in Sioux City.*

Dear Young Iowan:

If I were to give you a single gift, I would make it something real … something like a basketball. And not just any basketball—it would have to be one I used way back in the day. It may not have a lot of monetary value, but the sentimental value is priceless. At some point you'll be trying to decide whether or not to go out and hit the actual hard courts or stay inside and pound the Sony virtual courts. Hopefully, this ball, ratty as it is, will bounce you in the right direction.

I give you an old worn-out ball to remind you to get in the game. I know, I know—you're thinking I've totally lost cool points, that I'm getting ready to start a lecture. And I am, sort of. I'm just a little worried that in the world you're living in you're not really a participant.

Between iPods, video games, cell phones, and laptops, I fear you don't really have much time to get in the game. The fact is there's nothing that can compare to being on the court as an actual player. Nothing compares, honestly, to the buzzer sounding in your ear when you are pushing your body and mind to their natural limits … all for the pursuit of a real-life, real-time goal. Competing on a team also does so much for your character.

Good Sense from the Good Folks of Iowa

You learn how to work with others, how to communicate, how to plan for success, and how to bounce back from failure. Those are the very things you need to succeed in the game of life.

I didn't start playing basketball with this deep, philosophical stuff in mind; I simply played because it was fun. But it amazes me when I think of the lessons I learned as an Iowa high school All-Stater, a college All-American, and as a pro athlete. By wearing out the ball I mentioned above, I was able to play in or visit seven foreign countries and travel to nearly every state in the U.S. In fact, I've had opportunities to live in many of the places I've visited. But, time and time again, I have always come back to Iowa, where you're more likely to be invited into the game than you are where people don't care as much about having you in the game.

Obviously, my love for basketball, especially Iowa basketball, is deep. The game and the state I played it in, and for, have shaped my life. But the most important thing I've learned is to choose to play, to explore my limits in tangible, bodily ways. Whether you choose other sports, music, or the arts is largely irrelevant. I don't care if you wear out a ball, as I did, or blow out a trumpet or paint your brush bristleless ... just do it. Be a real-life participant—don't just play one on TV.

Yours on the hardwood,

Jan

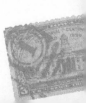

Craig Johnson

A Fort Dodge native and a graduate of Iowa Central Community College, Craig Johnson has been a mainstay in the lives of Iowa weather enthusiasts for nearly three decades. Currently the meteorologist for the Good Day Iowa *morning program on Fox28 television in Cedar Rapids, Iowa, his professional experience also includes twenty-seven years as a broadcast meteorologist in eastern Iowa for KWWL television in Waterloo and WMT-AM-FM-TV in Cedar Rapids. Johnson also writes two weekly weather columns for local newspapers:* Weather Whys Guy *and* Ag Weather.

A life-long science education enthusiast, Johnson makes numerous public appearances speaking to schools, civic groups, and professional organizations. A graduate of the University of Utah with a double major in meteorology and communications, Johnson has been the executive director of the Iowa Academy of Science since June of 2004.

Dear Young Iowan:

You and I have a lot in common. I am a native Iowan, having grown up in Fort Dodge during the 1950s and 1960s. My experiences were typical of many young Iowans at the time. I played on the banks of the Des Moines River, learned the value of money and hard work by carrying newspapers and working on the railroad. I breathed an atmosphere rich with family, friends, and neighbors.

Granted, Iowa has changed in the past forty years. There are fewer farms. Larger cities have grown while some smaller rural towns have diminished. We are more urban. But many of the same values that I grew up with are still with us today. One of the unsung gems of Iowa is access to the outdoors.

You might wonder why I consider our natural surroundings so important. My experiences taught me that stepping into natural spaces opened up an entirely new way of living. Not only was it relaxing, it renewed the spirit and opened my eyes to a world of plants, wildlife, landforms, and an expansive sky that instructed my own powers of observation. It catalyzed my career in science.

The trees, creeks, and hilly terrain surrounding the river of my youth put me in touch with nature nearly every day. A short ride on my bike would put me in open country where I had a great view of the sky in all directions. I learned to appreciate my surroundings while looking at the tiniest insects or looking for a huge, ominous thunderstorm threatening rain.

Iowa made it easy. Even in our biggest cities it takes only a matter of minutes to reach wide-open spaces. You can head to a park or just pull off to the side of a quiet road and you will be surrounded by tranquility.

The pace of life in Iowa helped direct my attention skyward. Fishing from or walking along a riverbank or a nearby woods caused me to develop a natural curiosity for everything around me. In the end it was the widening sky that drew my attention. By the age of ten, I was regularly looking out my bedroom window watching for lightning in the western sky. Winter blizzards captured my interest as I gradually transformed what many called "bad weather" into a hobby. I designed and built weather instruments and drafted weather maps. The in-your-face aspect of weather challenged me. I was learning to notice, think, and participate in scientific discovery.

Iowa, our nation, and our world need more scientists and more people who are able to work with technology, science, and mathematics. I can tell you that it doesn't require genius to become a scientist. It first requires an interest, an education, and, finally, a desire to put your skills and creativity to work.

Iowa offers the chance to develop all three. I encourage you to take the time to visit Iowa's outdoors and practice scientific method up close. State parks, forests and preserves are open for your benefit. Iowa's lakes, reservoirs, and rivers offer many outdoor opportunities. Go to libraries, bookstores, or access the Internet to learn more about our natural surroundings. Take that information into the field as you explore your surroundings.

For me, this scientific outlook led to a career as a broadcast meteorologist. I have helped countless people plan their work, recreation, and daily lives. I have forecast thunderstorms, tornadoes, blizzards, and, yes, even some mighty beautiful days. I have the weather to thank for putting me in touch with people and opportunities that I would have never dreamed possible.

So, through the lens of science, direct your gaze towards an ever-changing sky. Growing up well in Iowa means more than weathering the difficulties of youth, it means carefully appreciating the natural phenomena around you.

Your Weather Eye,

Craig Johnson

Interlude:
A Brief History of Iowa Letters and a Letter from the Editor, Zachary Michael Jack

Doctors advise against the reading of too many letters in one sitting, as they do against the overeating of popcorn, bonbons, and jelly beans. Kindly consider this interlude, then, a public service. Or fancy this: you've played the front nine and now you're in the clubhouse cooling your heels and reading some drivel left out on the table, *this* drivel.

Tomfoolery aside, be advised letters are serious business for my Iowa family. History reveals us to be a sanctimonious lot. Back in 1924, my great-aunt Mary Puffer, later to become Mary Brown, won a whopping $15.00 put up by a Mechanicsville, Iowa consortium of civic-minded, graybeard types for the best letter about Mechanicsville submitted to the *Pioneer Press*. In declaring my great-aunt Mary the prizewinner for her letter entitled "A Perfect Community," the Contest Committee wrote that they had a "bunch of good letters" but that one stood out as the cream of the crop. "The following letter," intoned the graybeards, "indicates a keen mind, close observation, and a fine mental attitude toward the home community." And either to register disbelief, to drive home a point, or both, the Committee added, "And it was written by a young person."

Aunt Mary died before I had a chance to ask whether she was simply flattering the Committee with her laudatory language—hoping to make a quick buck—or if, in fact, she intended sincere praise for her hometown, the Pork Capital of the World. An eighty-year-old letter deserves a bit of air, so here's an excerpt:

> I think it is possible to have a perfect community—at least a community as nearly perfect as anything has ever been. We have a splendid location for our little town of Mechanicsville amid Iowa's fertile soils; its lovely districts, its beautiful homes and flourishing farms. We have the finest location anywhere in Iowa—or anywhere

in the world for that matter, for most certainly Iowa is the best state
in the union and the best country in the world.

I think Mary would say that she meant those words sincerely. Mechanicsville was indeed, during those days, a bustling place fortuitously located on the coast-to-coast Lincoln Highway and the Chicago Northwestern rail line. McVille, as we called it, even boasted an opera house and the famed Page Motel, where Bob Hope and other stars overnighted. It saddens me to say that a mere sixty-five years after Mary caught the ears of our city fathers with her lyric lines, Iowa City journalist Osha Gray Davidson published a book, *Broken Heartland: The Rise of America's Rural Ghetto*, that opened with a case study on Mary's hometown, and mine. According to Davidson, the place had gone from riches to rags in the intervening six decades.

Or had we, its citizens?

Grant me this chicken and egg argument: Is it the letter that precedes a perfect community or the perfect community which elicits the letter? Do Iowa communities like Mechanicsville fall off their pedestal because they fail to inspire, or because their residents lose the ability to be inspired? In a nutshell, the question is this: who's to blame when love ends, the one who stops writing unrequited love letters or the one who is no longer sufficiently lovable to merit such gushing recitations? It won't surprise you that I think letters have the power to transform our relationships with one another and with the place we live, inasmuch as a letter alone can begin a courtship, sustain it, and end it.

My family has been writing love letters, mostly unrequited, to Iowa for years. We're still not sure if Iowa loves us back, and if she does, she gives us an awfully cold shoulder from December through March. My great-grandfather, Walter Thomas Jack, a farmer, teacher, and agricultural writer who published the soil conservation classic *The Furrow and Us* in 1946, loved our state dearly though he had no especially good reason to. He had been put up for adoption as a toddler, and though he had the good fortune—or poor fortune depending on how you look at it—to land with a stern family of Quakers, (the Jacks of West Branch, Iowa) his youth was far from orthodox and far from easy. True, West Branch was none too shabby a seedbed for good things, as Herbert Hoover and his family proved. But

West Branch in the 1880s and 1890s was a place of profound tragedy, as John and Margaret Jack lost their biological son, and Herbert Hoover lost his father to heart complications and his mother not long after. The Jacks and the Hoovers lived less than a mile apart, knew each other, and shared in one another's grief.

From the pieces of his memoirs that remain, it is safe to assume that Walter Jack was glad to marry Amber Pickert from Lisbon, Iowa in 1917, grateful to marry into a farm he could call his own and that he would till for the next half century. Walter's love letter to Iowa, less parochial than my Aunt Mary's, is no less superlative. In *The Furrow and Us*, he writes:

> My place is under Iowa skies, floored with the world's best soil and walled in by the emerald skyline of native oaks. I have planted and harvested these fertile fields for many years and have learned from mother nature that she holds no grudge. She has healed the wounds and scars I thoughtlessly made on her contour and patiently replaced the fertility I so lavishly spent.

Perhaps I bring to Walter's *Dear Iowa* a great-grandson's overly sensitive ears, but I hear both ingratitude and gratitude in this passage and elsewhere in *The Furrow and Us*. My hunch is strong that it took the writing of this letter and many like it, these effortful mid-life benedictions, to tilt the scales in favor of his thanksgiving. In Walter's case, as in so many others, it could have gone either way—bitterness and resentment at the poor hand dealt him or love and gratitude for the salvation he had known. In putting pen to paper in an open love letter to Iowa and to Mother Nature, he made his decision.

⧼⧽

Iowa has produced more than its fair share of famous and habitual letter writers, including, in our lifetime, the inimitable Ann Landers and Abigail Van Buren (Dear Abby) from Sioux City. To begin at the beginning of Iowa letters, though, it is necessary to resurrect the original Henry Wallace. "Uncle Henry," as he came to be known, prided himself on being on a familiar, first-namey basis with the loyal readers of his *Wallaces Farmer*. Good old Uncle Henry made no attempt to disguise his moralizing, appending the name "Uncle Henry's Sermons" to the letter-like epistles he wrote for *Wallaces*

Farmer. In one late nineteenth-century series, *Letters to the Farm Boy*, Good Ol' Uncle Henry explains to an imagined farmer's son—a "Young Iowan" if you will—his qualifications for writing: "Your Uncle Henry is now over sixty years old, and can, therefore talk to you as he would not have dared to do twenty years ago." In another letter on the subject of a farm boy and his temper, Wallace the Elder writes, "My Dear Boy: I have not sized you up as a goody-goody boy such as too often figure in the Sunday school books. Such boys are too often like the apples that ripen too early, indicating that the tree is on the decline."

Another famous Iowan fond of letters was Isaac Phillips Roberts, who moved to Iowa in 1862 with his young bride to take up farming in Mount Pleasant. Roberts proved a quick study as a pioneer farmer and, before the decade was through, he had been hired as a superintendent of the farm and secretary of the board of trustees of the newly formed Iowa Agricultural College at Ames—Iowa State University to you and me. In his book *The Fertility of the Land*, Roberts, like Wallace, invents a composite farm boy as a conversational foil. In a chapter subtitled "A Chat with a Young Farmer," Roberts writes:

> *I am well acquainted with you, though you are not acquainted with me, and being acquainted and older than you are, I cannot forbear entering into a little familiar chat. I know your thoughts, your toils and sorrows and discouragements; your aspirations, hopes and joys. I know, too, what fiber, endurance and patience farm work gives to the boys who make the most of what an outdoor life with nature has to offer. I know how hot it is in August under the peak of the flat-roofed barn, how large the forkfuls are that the stalwart pitcher thrusts into the only hole where light and air can enter. I know how high the thistles grow, and how far the rows of corn stretch out. I know, too, the freedom, fun and work of the old farm that make one expand, enjoy and grow, and leave no bitter memories. I know you well, my boy—how green and brown you feel when you come to the noisy city, and how you would like to be free and cool again!*

So it is that a little bit of success, or a lot in the case of Henry Wallace and Isaac Phillips Roberts, easily turns us into barnyard philosophers, speechifiers, and lay preachers. But how wonderful these letters are, and how wonderfully transparent. Of course Isaac Phillips Roberts writes as much for himself in the passage above as he does to the young farmer. When he writes "to be free and cool again!" it is as much to gratify his own boyhood nostalgia as it is to mind-read his conjured young farmer. To pretend otherwise of a letter—that is, that its audience is not as much the writer as the written—is to deny the full power of its expression.

Long live, then, the silly, awkward, profound letter! Where else do we find ourselves so much wiser and so much more tongue-tied than we ever imagined? When my Aunt Mary ascended the makeshift stage to receive her fifteen bucks from the Contest Committee, she was, *The Pioneer Press* reported, "profusely applauded." Would that we were all similarly rewarded for our hopelessly bigheaded, perfectly priceless letters.

Aunt Mary had discovered, in one fell swoop, the virtue and the vice of the open letter—its sweet sincerity on one hand, its terrific presumption on the other. In her last paragraph, her letter's grand finale, Miss Mary Puffer, still a teenager herself, writes to her peers:

> Before you are in high school you should see that you get more independent from your elders each day, that is, depending less on them for your support. Helping to support yourself is the stepping stone of supporting others. I believe that is the cause of so many bad results of young people today. They start too late in life to depend on themselves. You should learn to live for yourself first—experiment on yourself. Mother Nature is very wise, but failure to understand her in time has meant failure of many fine young lives. So, girls and boys should begin to take interest and to help in their community early in their life, and I promise it will pay.

So as not to be above all this nonsense, or below all this transcendence, I offer, in closing, my own, abbreviated letter, orphaned, as it is, from the rest of the collection. It is written, I must admit, in haste, but not without thought, and penned to young Iowans everywhere and, in particular, to my nephew Henry. Fitting, then, that I doff my cap to the elder Henry Wallace and sign it, naturally, "Uncle Zachary."

Dear Young Iowan:

Twilight tonight couldn't make up its mind. Last weekend Gran called it "messy," and she sat there, ninety-years-old in May, looking very satisfied with it, I guess because life is beautiful in a messy way. And when you're ninety you see it coming and you like it red and angry and cool and blue all at once.

Graduation is this Saturday and then I start teaching summer school, but don't feel sorry for me. Just one class and quite a bit more time knocking around home. I like how the hours swell in the summer, and I like days when the biggest decision is what to have for dessert: popsicle or ice cream. Lately, it's ice cream, hands down, sometimes out of a measuring cup, when the bowls get used up; other times straight out of the carton like a raccoon.

Each day when I have my "break" I go a different way out of town, though I never seem to go North, I guess because in the old maps the wind blows from up there, all icy and full of himself. If I have my druthers, I'll follow the sloughs south, out of town. Sometimes I stay on the blacktop going straight towards the river, but if it's not too hot I cross over onto the gravel road heading west. I like that one because it's flat until you get to the bridge, which is a good place to pause, pat yourself on the back for coming this far, and think cool, watery thoughts. Then it's straight uphill if you want to earn the view where the schoolhouse looks storybook.

On my way back this time, I had a red-winged blackbird on my case for at least a quarter of a mile. You ever had that happen? He put me in his crosshairs somewhere around the creek-crossing and wouldn't let go, screeching as if I had stolen his first-born. Face to face, a scorned red-wing looks like an angry headmaster or a sharp-beaked county clerk. But then they're scarier than that, too, those red-wings, and I don't suppose there's anything human to which to compare them. After suffering so many scoldings and sorties, you want to say "Alright already … I'm going. I'm going!"

After a half mile or so craning to see my attacker, my neck started hurting, so I kept track of the red wing's antics by following its shadow on the rock roadbed, a shadow all broken up, like a vulture's cast onto a canyon floor in some old Western. The bird-shadow looked like Batman for a bit, then like the angel of death. This bright, beautiful day and this dark, dark bird with flames for wings and that gravel road always like an afterlife—flat, flat, flat and the crest of the hill close but never getting any closer. What is it the Irish say in their blessing, *May the road rise to meet you?*

I'm still half-way looking for a new house, so maybe the next time you visit I'll answer at a new door. Sometimes I worry I'm too weary for the rigmarole of a new place ... all the back and forth, which I guess is what stops widows. It seems like no matter who you're mortgaged to you always end up calling some bright-eyed, bushy-tailed, twenty-something in Des Moines who is too glad to arrange for payment. I always wonder how they can stay so happy there in their cubicles. Probably it's the kind of happiness that comes when someone else is paying for the ink pens and air conditioning.

Country homes on paved roads fetch higher resale prices, it's true, but I'd actually like some dusty, graveled route like the one I grew up on. When you live on a rock road it's a little like sharing the block with a cranky old dog ... you and the neighbors know where to scratch it to keep it from biting but no one else does. Say what you will about gravel chewing up Goodyears and chipping clear coats, but it's a great way to keep the crowd from your door even if your ditch lilies do get dusty.

You can choose a husband or wife that way, too, by taking your forefinger and seeing how much dust is on them, like they do with coffee tables in furniture polish commercials. Usually the dustier the better.

Gravel roads remind me of how Grampy used to pick up rocks down on his hands and knees in the ditch, nit-picking. Seeing a farmer on his knees never did sit right with me. If you were picking up rocks with Grampy, you had to be sure to pick up anything bigger than a pea. With my dad, it was anything bigger than a marble, and by the time you're helping me pick rocks out of my ditch, I'll bring my forefinger and thumb together to make the universal symbol for "leave it, man, it's smaller than a quarter," which is also the universal symbol for a-okay and the universal peephole through which to view scary movies. Then we'll call it a day and have us some ice cream.

Ice cream breaks at midday . . . That's what older Iowans mean when they say the younger generation is going to hell in a handbasket.

I started my bike ride too late tonight and didn't get in until it was dark. I didn't meet too many cars on the road, thank goodness, but I did meet one of those high-rider platform sprayers, the ones that look like giant grasshoppers with their mean wings tucked back in attack mode. It was road-hogging. I couldn't see the man behind the machine, but I could see the sunset smeared all over his plate-glass window, and it was messy.

I wanted to ride right under him, like you sometimes see in the movies where a truck is gunning for the action hero and there's no way out until our hero lays flat on the ground and the truck passes right over him. Straight into the belly of the whale, I say.

Always, always do your own stunts.

Love and treachery,

Uncle Zachary

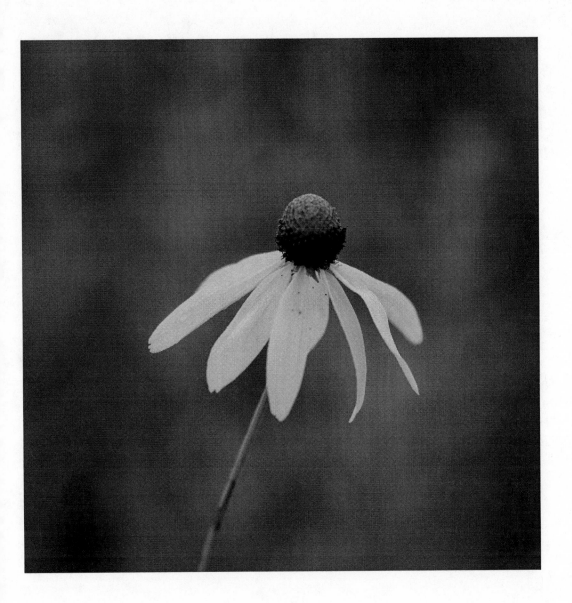

Photographs © Richard Sjolund

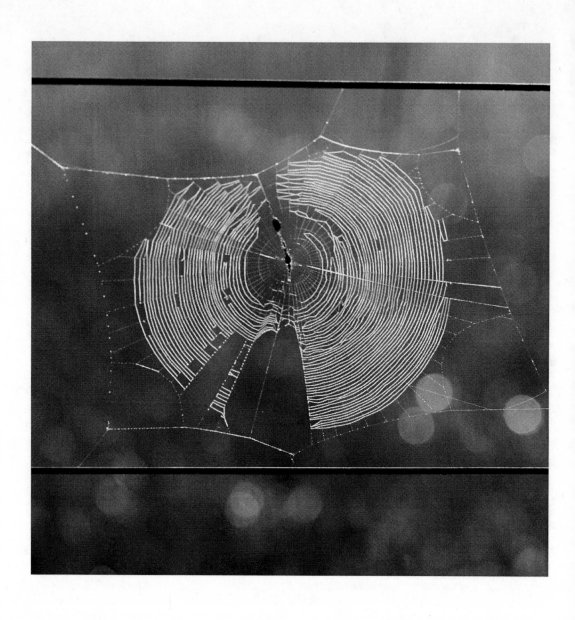

Letters to a Young Iowan, Part Two
Last Names K-Z

Jeffrey A. Kaufmann
Catfish Keith
Frederick L. Kirschenmann
Ted Kooser
Adrienne Lamberti
Nancy Landess
Michael Landorf
James A. Leach
Robert Leonard
Barbara Lounsberry
Bonnie Mansfield
Renee Mauser
Bill McAnally
Daniel McFarland
Steve McGuire
Karen Menz
Cornelia F. Mutel
Neil Nakadate
Marvin Negley
Jim Pease
Sally J. Pederson
Bob Peterson

Terry Pitts
John Price
Trent D. Reedy
Rachelle (Riki) H. Saltzman
Myrna Sandvik
Ron Sandvik
Sharon and Tom Savage
Robert Sayre
James Calvin Schaap
Nancy Schmidt
Susan Troutman See
Daniel H. Smith
Tracy Steil
Larry Stone
Rod Sullivan
Mary Swander
Sarah S. Uthoff
Christie Vilsack
Timothy Walch
Ed Williams
Kevin Woods

Good Sense from the Good Folks of Iowa

Jeffrey A. Kaufmann

Since birth Jeff Kaufmann has lived on a two hundred seventy-acre Iowa Century Farm that serves as headquarters for a twelve-hundred-acre farming operation producing crops, cattle, hogs, sheep, and poultry. Elected to the Iowa House of Representatives in 2004 from District 79, Kaufmann's perspective is dynamically local: he is actively involved in local community service and historical preservation, including posts as the president of the Wilton community school board and chairman of the Sugar Creek Township Board of Trustees.

Kaufmann, who earned undergraduate as well as graduate degrees from the nearby University of Iowa, edits the half-century old Cedar County Historical Review, *a publication that has earned the Peterson-Harlan Award from the State Historical Society of Iowa. Kaufmann, who is a professor of history at Muscatine Community College, lives with his wife, Vicki, and their three sons, Robert, Jacob, and John. They remain on the banks of Sugar Creek with no plans of leaving.*

Dear Young Iowan:

I would so much like to freeze my boyhood and hand it to you as an everlasting gift.

I am the seventh-generation to live by Sugar Creek in southern Cedar County in eastern Iowa. When I was growing up along those banks, every day was an adventure: another stream to follow to its source, another forest to traverse, another friend from town to show the wonders of the county. I can't ever remember a day of being bored. And the seasons are so pronounced in my little corner of heaven.

I still smell and feel home when I am in the chamber of the House of Representatives in Des Moines. In fact, I'll share a secret with you—I have often "gone home" during a long tirade of political rhetoric. I go home to the smell of April and new life, a cool breeze on a summer evening, the sheer beauty of an oak timber in October, and the stillness of a snow-covered pasture. I still hear my mother calling me home to a feast awaiting her hungry little explorer. And I will forever remember my father's eyes when he gazed at a field of fresh cut hay or a new fence, straight as an arrow, or the corn just breaking the soil after a slow drenching rain. That gaze, the

Good Sense from the Good Folks of Iowa

pride and satisfaction it contained, is the key to our attachment to the land, and our attachment to the land is, in turn, the key to our success.

By far the greatest gift of all will be the sight of future generations, weary and maybe anxious, finding home again after long absence. Home may be different fifty years from now, but the power of place will remain.

The feeling of contentment that I pray all of you experience should not be counted in awards or dollars, but, instead, in the sense of a job well-done and the possibility of an adventure calling as close as just outside your door.

In today's world full of diversions—a time when you can travel anywhere in the world in a variety of ways—you have to be deliberate about finding your corner of heaven on the banks of a creek like Sugar Creek. But when you find it—that rippling water and those seasons, those voices from your past will never leave you—listen. There may be fewer places to really listen now, but they are still there. I suggest the haymow in the big red barn on a rainy day or the timber along the creek just north of the lime kilns or one of the many country cemeteries where your ancestors rest.

If you don't quite understand me now, keep listening, and one day it will become crystal clear. When it does, come and let me know, will you? The joy of that day will just about complete my corner of heaven.

You have my most important prayer.

Love,

Jeff Kaufmann

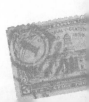

Catfish Keith

Catfish Keith is an internationally known blues singer, songwriter, and bottleneck slide guitarist, and has been based out of the Iowa City area for nearly twenty years. In 1990, Catfish and his manager and wife, Penny Cahill, formed their own record label, Fish Tail Records, and have released ten number-one-charting solo albums, some of which have been nominated for the prestigious W. C. Handy Blues Award for the best acoustic blues album. Catfish has headlined thousands of concerts and music festivals around the globe and has appeared with Ray Charles, John Lee Hooker, Bonnie Raitt, B.B. King, Leo Kottke and many, many others.

Dear Young Iowan:

This is to all the young dreamers, especially musicians and creative artists of every stripe.

I write this to encourage you to pursue your dreams.

Here's my story: As a teenager, I got captivated by the sounds of the acoustic guitar, and thirty years, ten albums, thousands of gigs, and dozens of international tours later, I'm still following that very same dream.

I've made my lifestyle and living totally from playing guitar and singing. My focus has been on the great American treasure trove of blues and roots music.

Our travels from my music career have taken us all over the world, touring through all of the U.S.A., the Caribbean, Canada, the U.K., Ireland, Europe, and Asia. We continue to make Iowa our home. It's where my wife and I grew up and where our families live.

I was born in East Chicago, Indiana. When I was six or so, my family moved to Davenport, Iowa, where I finished high school in 1979. I had been heavily involved in choir, plays, and musicals. At age fourteen I started playing guitar, and my imagination and soul were transported by the sounds of solo, acoustic guitar and the Delta blues, slide and fingerpicking guitar that sounded like a whole orchestra or band all by itself.

The legacy is deep and it's a tradition of innovation that I've been honored to continue. The music has been called many things—folk music,

135

country blues, acoustic blues, roots music, island music; it's broad based and includes a wide variety of sounds. The main connector is that it's all a very real, heartfelt, soulful, and individual expression, where one person can make the whole sound by playing bass, melody, harmony, rhythm, and singing and stomping all at the same time. I love it!

What I'm saying is that once you have found your passion in life, stick to it. Mine is music, yours could be any artistic pursuit. Once I found it, it was a revelation, and there was no question in my mind that that's what I absolutely wanted to do, and I became very determined to do it.

The way I did it myself was my own path; you have to find your own path yourself and have a singular devotion to it. Once I knew what I wanted to do, it lit up a new creative fire within. I spent hours and hours every day, listening and absorbing and teaching myself hundreds of songs and licks and techniques. I'd listen close to records (no CDs back then!), and try to make my own version of what I heard. I'd learn by watching other players, and in some cases absorbing the knowledge firsthand from heroes and legendary players like Leo Kottke, Honeyboy Edwards, Homesick James, Johnny Shines, Jessie Mae Hemphill, Libba Cotten, Greg Brown and so many others. The eventual result was my own style.

In my late teens and early twenties, I took to the road, seeing what there was to see. It was a great period of exploration and learning. I had a rusty 1973 Oldsmobile that I lived in, doing gigs wherever I could. I spent years traveling throughout every corner of the continent. I spent a couple of winters living in the Virgin Islands too, living on a sailboat for a while, inspired by a wealth of island music that added a new dimension to my tunes. I was never rich with money, but I was rich with experience. I never had to have a "real" job; I was always able to scrape enough together to enjoy life, and make it to the next gig.

The main thing is to absorb everything, learn everything you can, then take it all to *be yourself*. Everybody copies at first—absolutely nothing comes from a vacuum. This applies to music, art, writing, inventing. The wonderful thing I found in the guitar was an instrument that is reinvented over and over. Most everybody has their individual style within them, just waiting to come out. You have yours within you. The excitement and fulfillment from this is very rich and rewarding. If you are lucky and determined and have a talent for it, you will take it as far as your dreams can take you.

Yours truly,

Catfish Keith

Frederick L. Kirschenmann

A native of North Dakota, Frederick L. Kirschenmann has devoted much of his adult life to sustainable farming in Iowa, particularly in his role as director for the Aldo Leopold Center for Sustainable Farming at Iowa State University.

Kirschenmann Family Farms, one of the first to be certified organic in 1980, has been part of a number of research studies and has been featured in national publications including National Geographic, Smithsonian, Audubon, Business Week, Los Angeles Times, *and* Gourmet. *In 2001 Kirschenmann received the Seventh Generation Research Award from the Center for Rural Affairs for his work in sustainable food and farming systems. He was also named a 2002 Leader of the Year in Agriculture by* Progressive Farmer *publications.*

Dear Young Iowan:

I am seventy-one years old—you are eight—and I have been sitting here trying to figure out how to start this conversation.

I am overcome with sadness because of the harm we have done to the world that you are about to inherit. According to a recently released United Nations report, produced by fourteen hundred scientists, we have succeeded in so degrading the air, water, and climate of this wonderful planet we call home that the long-term well-being of humans is now threatened.

We did all of this in just the past fifty years! And we seem incapable of changing our ways while there is still time to turn things around. So I have to face the fact I am part of a generation that is going to hand over a world to you that, for the first time since our species has appeared, may not be habitable. What can I say?

The irony is that none of us intended to do this. In fact we only wanted a better world for you and all the generations to follow. We were so successful at creating a succession of new tools to make life better, more convenient, more enjoyable, and safer that we forgot to pay attention to the many unintended consequences of all of our inventions.

We were euphoric when we found that we could drive powerful machines with cheap energy when we discovered coal and oil and natural gas. Our machines, driven by cheap energy, enabled us to build wonderful homes, drive impressively fast cars, fly sleek airplanes, grow unimaginable amounts of food. We began to envision a human-designed and human-created utopia in which we could all live happily ever after.

And all the while we did not realize that we were eroding our precious soils, reducing your future capacity to produce food, pushing tons of carbon dioxide into the air only to start a long, irreversible process of global warming that will disrupt the relatively stable climates we have enjoyed, and making many of our bodies of water uninhabitable for the abundant sea life that is part of the foundation of this incredibly productive, vibrant planet.

But, for a little while, we still have time to turn things around, and I pledge myself to join with you and all of the wonderful new generation of young people in Iowa and around the world who are now committing themselves to a different future—a future in which we are determined to clean up our messes, to insure that air and water and soil and all of life on the planet are used so that the planet's health—its capacity for self-renewal—is enriched, not diminished. I pledge myself to do everything I can to stop the insane notion that "progress" is living high on the hog and ignoring the fact that continuing to do so will slowly kill us. I pledge myself to do this so that you, and the generations that follow you, can live in a world of more life rather than more things.

Together we can do this.

With love,

Frederick Kirschenmann

Good Sense from the Good Folks of Iowa

Ted Kooser

The former poet laureate of the United States, Ted Kooser was born in Ames and lived there through his college years at Iowa State University, after which he taught high school in Madrid, Iowa for one year. Though Kooser has made a home in Nebraska during disparate careers as an insurance executive, writer, and professor at the University of Nebraska, he maintains strong Iowa roots. His mother's parents lived in Guttenberg, a town which Kooser has written about frequently.

A favorite on both National Public Radio and CBS's Sunday Morning, *Kooser has published more than ten books, two with essayist and short story writer Jim Harrison. Called a "thoroughly American poet" by former poet laureate Billy Collins, Kooser is married to Kathleen Rutledge, the editor of the* Lincoln Journal Star.

Dear Young Iowan:

Lots of young people are angry about this and that, and there's nothing wrong with anger, but I'd like to recommend that you balance your anger with kindness. Most of the people you'll encounter are doing the best they can, trying to live good lives, sometimes against great odds—ignorance, prejudice, intolerance, and so on—and you can help to make the world a better place by being kind to them. We need a lot more kindness, and you can contribute.

There's never a good excuse for being mean to anyone.

Ted Kooser

Adrienne Lamberti

Adrienne Lamberti grew up on an Iowa Century Farm—Silver Valley Farms in Norwalk—where she helped with the corn, soybean, and alfalfa crops and a herd of milking shorthorn dairy cattle.

Lamberti holds an MA in creative writing and a PhD in rhetoric and professional communication, both from Iowa State University, where she taught business communication and technical writing. Currently, Lamberti coordinates the professional writing program at the University of Northern Iowa, where she teaches courses including document design, editing, and technical communication. Having witnessed many misreadings of Jonathan Swift's "A Modest Proposal," Lamberti wishes to caution the reader upfront that the two letters to a young Iowan that follow—from the imaginary LDE University and its vice president "John D. Smith"—are purely fictional and purposefully satirical. The letters' typography, distinct from the rest of this volume, is intended to heighten the parody.

LDE University
Tempe, Arizona

Young Iowan
Des Moines, Iowa

Dear **Young Iowan**:

Congratulations! This letter serves as notification of your acceptance[1] into Long Distance Education University, the nation's premier online university. LDE serves many college students in **Iowa** who wish to accelerate their educational experience. In fact, most teachers throughout America recognize LDE's name!

No more sitting in stuffy classrooms, worrying that the state of **Iowa** legislature will again slash educational funding, or encountering professors from diverse cultures.[2] With LDE's college program, you'll never have to personally interact with any professors at all! How great is that?

At LDE, we realize that "learning for the sake of learning" is out of fashion. Today's college student isn't interested in paying his hard-earned money[3] for an education; today's college student wants a <u>degree</u>. In this country, a college degree guarantees that you can achieve your career dreams. That's why LDE's mission is to help each student reach his full human potential as a member of the American work force.

Good Sense from the Good Folks of Iowa

Unlike the average nonprofit university, LDE is a member of American industry—we understand how business really works. When it comes to courses in the liberal arts, fine arts, cultural issues, politics, etc., LDE will help you jump through those hoops as quickly as possible, so you can focus on the classes that matter to employers.[4]

But you probably know all of this—that's why you applied to our program. You've already accomplished the hardest step; now, all you have to do is take the classes! Once LDE receives your first tuition payment, we'll send you the username and password necessary for logging in to our website and registering for courses. The enclosed pamphlet will guide you through this easy process.[5]

Finally, now that you're a real college student, tell the world with LDE's line of sportswear! Our website includes special prices on shirts, sweats, mugs, shot glasses, and more. And be sure to talk to your friends about LDE; if you submit their email addresses to our website, we'll send them information about our program.

Once again, **Young Iowan**, congratulations! Long Distance Education University is revolutionizing higher education in the state of **Iowa**, and your wise decision to become a part of our program means that you, too, are contributing to this exciting change.

Sincerely,

John D. Smith

John D. Smith
Vice President of Admissions
LDE University

[1] Upon successful processing of your first tuition check, official notification of acceptance into our program will be mailed to you.

[2] Note: Assignments that cannot be evaluated via LDE's electronic servers are graded at our satellite campus in New Delhi, India.

[3] Remind your father that he can receive a tax break for his financial contributions to your tuition!

[4] LDE is working to serve its students by securing accreditation for our courses.

[5] Questions? Call our toll-free number Monday-Friday, 9 a.m.-5 p.m. Pacific.

LDE University
Tempe, Arizona

Young Iowan
Des Moines, Iowa

Dear **Young Iowan**:

Can you believe only a month has passed since you've joined Long Distance Education University, the nation's premier online university? Now that your first tuition check has been processed, you are officially enrolled in LDE. Congratulations! In this letter, you'll find your username and password for logging on to our website and registering for courses.

Family. It's important. And we want you, **Young Iowan**, to know that you're a member of the LDE family. We'll be there as you strive to meet your goals for the future. Yes, we promise the personalized support so essential for achieving success in today's fast-paced world.[6]

At LDE, we realize that you want to support your family, too. And now it's easier than ever! Simply check the "endowment" box on your next tuition statement and show everyone that you, too, will always be there for your family.[7]

You also can show your family pride with LDE's line of sportswear! Our website includes special prices on shirts, sweats, mugs, shot glasses, and more. And be sure to talk to your friends about LDE; if you submit their email addresses to our website, we'll send them information about our program. With your help, the LDE family will become even bigger and better!

Once again, **Young Iowan**, congratulations on becoming a member of the LDE family, and taking the first step towards an exciting future!

Sincerely,

John D. Smith

John D. Smith
Vice President of Admissions
LDE University

[6]See our website for instructions on adding your email address to our LDE listserv!
[7]Checking the "endowment" box acts as authorization for enrollment in the LDE Family Giving Program.

Good Sense from the Good Folks of Iowa

Nancy Landess

A graduate of Drake University, Nancy Landess manages the tourism office of the Iowa Department of Economic Development. She is responsible for developing and implementing programs that support and promote Iowa's tourism opportunities for economic growth. Landess started with the Iowa Department of Economic Development in 1977 and has served as the manager of the tourism office since September 1995. She is the past chair of the National Council of State Tourism Directors (NCSTD) and received the State Tourism Director of the Year award in 2004. She is the past chair of the multi-state promotional organizations Mississippi River Country and America's Heartland.

Dear Young Iowan:

I know you are busy and involved in lots of activities. But I want to encourage you to take time to experience Iowa. I also want to share some suggestions with you on what I think makes our state so special.

Iowa is blessed with great natural beauty. Bordered by America's two greatest rivers, the Missouri and the Mississippi, Iowa boasts two National Scenic Byways with the Great River Road and the Loess Hills Scenic Byway. Did you know you will only find loess soil at the depths you will see in western Iowa in one other place in the world: China?

Our state is home to three national immigrant museums. The Vesterheim Norwegian-American Museum in Decorah, the National Czech and Slovak Museum and Library in Cedar Rapids, and the Danish Immigrant Museum in Elk Horn share rich stories of our history and heritage. The Amana Colonies celebrate their German roots while Pella and Orange City honor their Dutch heritage. You will learn a lot about their traditions by visiting these communities.

Sometimes it is fun to travel with your grandparents. Here are some ideas that you might enjoy with them. The National Mississippi River Museum and Aquarium in Dubuque is the only national interpretive center for the Mississippi where you can see live animals from the river, including an alligator. Next door is Iowa's first indoor water park. The Science Center of Iowa in Des Moines features interactive galleries and has an IMAX theater.

Matchstick Marvels in Gladbrook displays detailed models and sculptures made entirely of wooden matchsticks. Do you like ice cream? Try some at the Ice Cream Capital of the World Visitor Center in Le Mars. And, we have the world's largest popcorn ball in Sac City that is seven-feet tall and weighs 3,100 pounds!

Do you go to the movies? You can visit movie sites in Iowa. In Dyersville, you will find the *Field of Dreams*, where you can run the bases, play catch, or cheer from the bleachers. The *Bridges of Madison County* was also filmed in Iowa, and you can tour the covered bridges featured in the movie. Winterset is in Madison County, so, while you are there, tour the birthplace of the movie actor John Wayne.

You can't miss the Iowa State Fair! It is held annually in August and draws over one million people. See the famous butter cow and treat yourself to almost any food on a stick. Be sure to stop in the Iowa Tourism Building during the fair and learn more about all there is to see and do in our state.

It's fun to plan a trip around a theme. How about sports? It would include a stop at the Bob Feller Museum in Van Meter. Feller had a Hall of Fame baseball career with the Cleveland Indians. Iowa has the only museum in the world dedicated to sprint car racing. Knoxville is home to the Sprint Car Museum and Hall of Fame and hosts the Knoxville Nationals every August. The National Motorcycle Museum and Hall of Fame is in Anamosa. Iowa is home to the International Wrestling Museum. The Hall of Pride in Des Moines invites all schools in the state to highlight their educational system and extracurricular activities. There you can take your turn at being an umpire calling balls and strikes, or try your hand at being a sports announcer.

I know you'll get hungry during your travels in Iowa. Why not try a unique local restaurant? We call it culinary tourism, but you'll just call it great Iowa food. Breitbach's Country Dining, located in Balltown, is Iowa's oldest restaurant. They have good food and great pie! Maytag blue cheese is made in Iowa, and you can visit the cheese plant near Newton. As you travel in the state, look for the locally-owned restaurants and cafes. You can always have some fast food when you get back home.

If you like music, you should really visit the River Music Experience in Davenport and learn about the music from up and down the Mississippi

River. Davenport also offers the Bix Biederbecke Jazz Festival each July to celebrate jazz music made famous by their native son. Be sure to visit Music Man Square in Mason City to learn about Meredith Willson, who was born and raised there. Glenn Miller was born in Clarinda and that community hosts a festival every year featuring the big band sound.

Did you know that artist Grant Wood was from Iowa? You can visit the American Gothic House in Eldon. Take your pitchfork and have your photo taken in front of the house. You can see many paintings by Grant Wood at the Cedar Rapids Museum of Art and the Figge Museum of Art in Davenport.

While you are traveling the state, look for our state symbols. These include the wild rose as our state flower, eastern goldfinch as our state bird, oak trees as our state tree and the geode as our state rock. I also encourage you to visit our state capitol in Des Moines. It features a 275-foot, gold-leafed dome, five-story law library, scale model of Battleship Iowa and a collection of First Lady dolls. While you are in Des Moines, take time to visit Terrace Hill, home to the Governor and a National Historic Landmark.

There is so much that makes Iowa special. Have fun!

Sincerely,

Nancy

Michael Landorf

A one-time torpedoman in the U.S. Navy now working for the Iowa Department of Transportation, Michael Landorf is as dynamic on the page as off. After graduating from high school in Independence and attending Loras College in Dubuque and Mankato State University in Mankato, Minnesota, Landorf began his Navy service in Hawai`i.

Landorf's ecstatic nature carries over into his marriage to his wife Beverly, who he describes, in e. e. cummings fashion, as a "bodaciouslybeautifulbabe" and to his work as a poet in his previously self-published collections outskirts of town *and* from a different direction *as well as in a soon-to-be-released third compilation. Landorf is also passionately devoted to his children and his grandsons, Blayke and Marcus, with whom he enjoys gathering native medicines and attending powwows. Ever the experimental prose-poet, Landorf, who spells his name* michaelandorf *for poetic occasions, blends letter writing and poetry writing in his message to a young Iowan.*

Dear Young Iowan:

> young iwanian, each generation
> seems to alienate itself
> further and further from nature
> which results in too many people being separated from the
>   natural world
> for we must each realize
> that everything we eat and drink and breathe
> is created by a balanced ecosystem existing & swirling around us
> each of us as a human being
> should have one hand outstretched reaching towards the sky
> and one hand touching the earth mother
> to coexist with the spiritual world
> and to reattach to our transplanted roots
> as Joseph Campbell once said in his book *The Power of Myth*
> quoting the Upanishads:
> "When before the beauty of a sunset or of a mountain you pause and
>   exclaim,
> 'Ah,' you are participating in divinity."

it has been said that everything we do in life
is either a miracle or a crime
a curse or a blessing
so that ultimately we become either miraclemakers or criminals
doing social good or social harm
one should constantly be saying "god bless" out of appreciation &
        gratitude
rather than the words of condemnation spoken out of blind
        anger or fear

all religions are based on humanitarianism
while atheism is based on selfishness
without human kindness and benevolence there is no true happiness
do not wish for excess materialism and power
wish for good health and love in abundance
mankind's constant worship and obsession
for money is a form of modern-day idolatry
do not associate with toxic people
or those that are racists or pessimists or hypocrites
they will drag you down faster than you can ever lift them up
and always be a friend to those that are in need of a friend

in your lifetime
open your heart & home and dining table
as a meeting place for all races and religions
let your home be a wateringhole in a world that thirsts for wisdom
        & knowledge
be close to all the creatures that surround you
admit to being a treehugger … chipmunklover … weedkisser …
        dewsipper
rainbowchaser … rockrubber … windsniffer … toadstoolworshipper

experience a daily communion with nature
grow a garden and lawn
without herbicides or pesticides

set a good example rather than try to change anyone
as Martin Luther once said "sin bravely"
then you always have much to be forgiven for
we all must sin to be saved
we all must get sick to get well
accept your humanness as one of your finest mortal gifts
each of us in our own way are very fragile and frail and vulnerable

never stop dreaming
never let anyone steal your imagination & power
think in poetry
let romance rule your heart
learn to never take yourself too seriously
dance and sing to your own revolution
remember god and the angels love to laugh
so give them something to laugh about
believe in magic and the land of make-believe
in leprechauns and fairies and trolls and imaginary friends
smooch your own secret blarney stone
become a long-winded storyteller
make all the daily lives of those you deeply love
easier not harder
try hard not to break anyone's heart or let anyone break yours
be proud to finish last and humble if you must be first
always let the elders and children walk in front of you
(the turtle can outlive the rabbit by 399 years)

discover your muse before it has to pursue you
find a manitou in everything you consider holy
tap gently into your own inspiration
anoint yourself a secret spiritual name
plant ten trees for every one you cut down
plant ten flowers for every one you pick
say *no* ten times more than you utter the word *yes*
compliment ten times more than you criticize

love ten times more than you think you are loved
forgive tenfold more than you are forgiven

remember that your greatest teachers
are often those that dislike you
as Joseph Campbell said
"Love thine enemies because they are the instruments of your destiny."
they become your petty tyrants
who test your weaknesses rather than your strengths
who ultimately teach you who not to be like
rather than who to be like

be like the American Indians
and believe every day is the sabbath
listen to god who often speaks to us through silence
pray for those who you don't think are praying for you
prayer is one of the greatest powers in the universe
as a future parent or grandparent let prayer be a safety net
for your children and grandchildren's safety

—michaelandorf

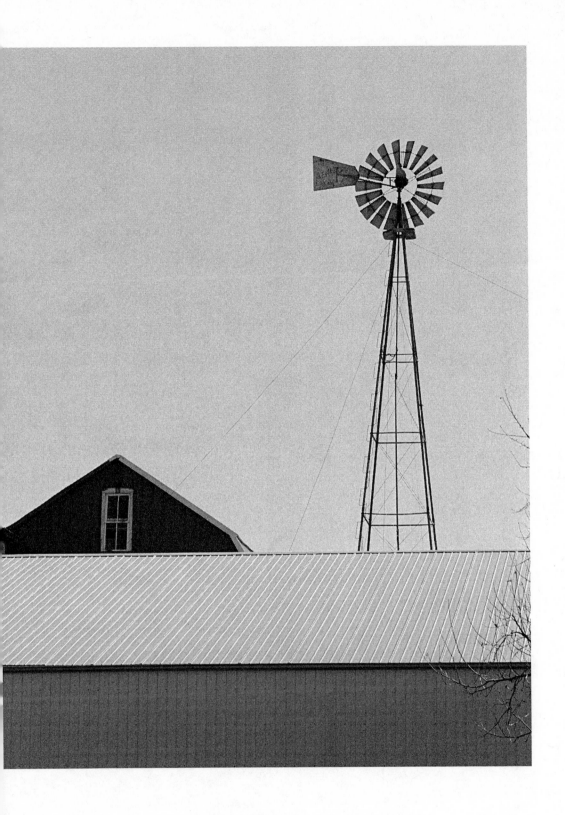

Photographs © Rod Strampe

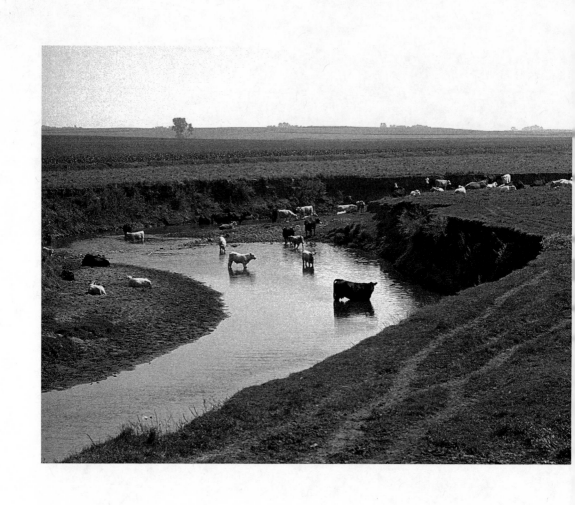

James A. Leach

Jim Leach represented Iowa honorably in the U.S. House of Representatives from 1976 to 2006. His former House assignment on the Committee on International Relations reflects his deep experience in foreign affairs dating back to his tenure as a foreign service officer in 1968 and 1969. Leach's resumé also includes work as a foreign service officer assigned to Arms Control and Disarmament Agency as a delegate to the United Nations General Assembly in 1971 and 1972—work that established a pattern of service to the U.N. that would earn Leach the Congressional Award for Commitment to the Principles of the U.N. Charter.

A recipient of honorary degrees from a half dozen colleges and universities, Jim Leach earned a BA in political science from Princeton University and an MA in Soviet politics from the School of Advanced International Studies at Johns Hopkins University. Born and raised in Davenport, Leach was a member of the Davenport High School football and wrestling teams, earning a State wrestling championship in 1960 and, later, election to the Wrestling Hall of Fame in Stillwater, Oklahoma and the International Wrestling Hall of Fame in Iowa. Leach and his wife, Elisabeth, and their children, Gallagher and Jenny, make their home in Iowa City.

Dear Young Iowan:

Intergenerational advice is suspect. This is because generational differences have never been greater and because your elders have not managed change as well as they might.

So let me simply note current phenomena and ask that you keep them in mind. The first is acceleration of change. Up to three or four generations ago, young people had few choices in life. Virtually everyone made their living doing exactly what their parents and grandparents did. The same could be said for matchmaking. Young people married only within their neighborhoods, and parents frequently determined who their spouses would be.

Today's explosion of choice is the wonder of our times. It is invigorating, but it is also discombobulating. Many choices exist between two or more positives; others involve temptations best avoided.

In your parents' generation and all generations that came before, a fundamental mantra was "learn from your mistakes." The truth of this advice may be eternal but, from your generation forward, it is not wise enough. Your task is still more profound: you must learn from the mistakes others make. For instance, modern drugs are so addictive that succumbing to temptation once or twice can lead to a lost life. When second chances don't exist, a young person has no choice except to learn from the consequences of the foibles of others.

At the societal level, weapons of mass destruction have been developed of such magnitude that their unleashing can destroy all civilization. In the history of man virtually every generation has known war. But, as Einstein noted, splitting the atom changed everything except our way of thinking. Because second chances may not exist, the next generation of leaders must help bring war itself under control.

Confucius observed several millennia ago that harmony within a family leads to harmony within society, within the nation, and between nations. It is harmony—respect for others, for nature, and for the environment— that must be inculcated in our lives. Harmony implies good values as well as individual and social discipline—the wisdom to do good and avoid temptations that are not love-driven.

In a big world with big obligations, the key is to learn from the mistakes of friends as well as elders. Respect, too, what they have done right. Don't be afraid to lead.

Sincerely,

James A. Leach

Robert Leonard

Robert Leonard was born in Des Moines in 1954. He graduated from Johnston High School in 1972 and the University of Northern Iowa in 1977. He received his MA in 1983 and PhD in 1986 from the University of Washington, Seattle in anthropology. He worked for the Zuni tribe in New Mexico from 1984 to 1987, when he joined the anthropology faculty at the University of New Mexico. He taught there until 2005, when it came time to come home.

Leonard is currently a partner in the anthropological consulting firm Human Inquiry, and is the author of Yellow Cab, *as well as dozens of anthropological papers and books. He currently lives with his wife Annie and their children, Asa and Johanna, on a farm south of Knoxville, Iowa.*

Dear Young Iowan:

I have known a great many Iowans in my day. They include a man who built great sailing ships over a century ago, a homecoming queen with a beautiful smile and polio, a sculptor who uses butter as her medium, a hooker who works the streets of Des Moines because she doesn't believe in welfare, a reformed drunk and truck driver who found God and became Governor and might have been President, a 20-year-old friend who I wish had talked to me before he hung himself in 1974, a 65-year-old woman from Pleasantville who seems 16 when I look into her eyes, a retired merchant marine who changes the world one letter to the editor at a time, an old man in an engineer's cap who makes ropes at county fairs so children can learn the old ways, a man who washes chicken heads down a drain in Waterloo, enough Olympic medalists and All-Americans in wrestling to fill a bus, a cattleman from Oskaloosa who believes that cows belong in green pastures and not feedlots, a mayor who lies awake at night trying to figure out how to bring an ethanol or switchgrass plant to his town, a single mom who homeschools nine kids in a trailer with the guidance of God, a gentle man who loved Appaloosas and blew his brains out when his wife left him, a book-loving doctor with four unpublished novels in a drawer at home who will write forever, a woman who teaches children of all ages how to ride bicycles at the state hospital in Woodward, a woman who buys organic produce for Hy-Vee who believes going organic is liberal nonsense, a boy in Ritalin chains, a man on TV with a dog puppet, a philosopher from Sioux City who believes that you and I exist only to serve as background to his own existence, a professor from Iowa City who teaches the world about Neanderthals, a man who chose to study criminology and social work in college after his little sister was murdered when he was 14, a sniper in Vietnam burdened with images that flip through his mind day and night like a slideshow, a former wrestler at UNI who teaches cowboy poetry at a university in Arizona, a couple who danced the night away at the Surf Ballroom in Clear Lake the night Buddy Holly, Ritchie Valens, and the Big Bopper crashed and died, that same couple who cried together the next morning, changed forever, a farmer who knew the world had gone to hell when hay bales got too big for one man to lift, a 60ish woman who played half-court girls basketball on the guard side of the court who could still cover Kobe better than half the NBA, a car thief from Keokuk, a concrete salesman whose face beams when he's told his adopted daughter looks just like him, a girl who pours beer in a small town bar who thinks we don't know that she has a meth problem, a heating and cooling man who collects Corvettes and ex-wives, a young man who chooses to build an elaborate and successful existence for himself on MySpace.com rather than in the real world, an old carpenter with big knuckles, a gruff demeanor, and a huge heart, a fallen lawyer who picked himself up and found success on the sales floor at the Home Depot in Ames, a young man fighting in Iraq, a gentle and forgiving Lutheran minister who wrote beautiful poetry for us all, and another who took lascivious pleasure in looking down from the pulpit and scolding generations of us for being sinners, a time traveler from the 60s still drinking Boone's Farm wine and smoking ditchweed, a television newswoman so focused on work she lives in a dumpy hotel in Urbandale, a successful restaurateur whose parents came from Mexico fifty years ago to pick sugar beets near Mason City, a successful restaurateur whose parents came from Italy a century ago to mine coal in West Des Moines, a man I suspect murdered his brother, the first black president of a national bar association, five cops who beat a man down with nightsticks in an alley, a man who cheats at cribbage, a trumpeter in the Navy band, and a former priest still saving souls and fighting for you and me and our way of life even as they toss him in jail for protesting, as well as thousands of other Iowans who take what life gives them and then make choices.

So, in closing, those are some of the thousands of Iowans I have known. I hope that I will know many more. Maybe even you.

So I'll say to you, don't be dumb or lazy or selfish or think that you are better than other people. Be thoughtful, get advice, try to choose wisely, and when you occasionally fall (and you will), get up, apologize profusely, figure out what it was you needed to learn, and start over. Seek adventure, have fun, work hard, and do good work. Look for love, and when you find it, hold its warm and tender hand in your own, gently.

Best wishes,

Robert Leonard

Barbara Lounsberry

Barbara Lounsberry was born and raised in Iowa. She has written books on literature and writing, and, in the 1990s, had the fun of editing three mystery novels set in Iowa, with each chapter written by a different Iowa author. The first novel, Time and Chance, *revolves around riverboat gambling; the second,* 16,000 Suspects: A RAGBRAI Mystery, *is set during Iowa's famous bicycle ride across the state.* Politics is Murder, *the third detective novel, is set during the Iowa governor's race in 2002.*

Dear Young Iowan:

My wish is that you flourish—and to that end I must alert you to a strange "atmospheric condition" that pervades the Great Plains. I speak of the midwestern climate of reserve, our quiet culture.

Perhaps you've never noticed this climate, this front that never leaves. Do fish notice the water in which they swim? Yet becoming aware of our regional (and statewide) legacy of reserve and developing strategies to deal with it can rightly be considered your first steps toward success—steps that will make all other successes possible.

But surely, you say, all Iowans aren't reserved. We all know people—some in our own families—who never stop talking! We wish they would talk *less*. But, during the Great Iowa Flood of 1993, *USA Today* headlined an article "Midwest Stoic as Floods Finally Ebb," and in 1996, reporters wrote this about presidential candidate Bob Dole's Russell, Kansas hometown: "This is a place that reveres plain, blunt speech; jokes that sound like insults; and stoic endurance." There's that *stoic* again.

A couple years ago when North Dakotans thought the word "North" gave a chilly impression and wanted to drop it and become just "Dakota," Texas columnist Molly Ivins visited and observed: "'Just Dakotans'" are not given to easy chat. The whole state still believes Loose Lips Sink Ships."

A bit closer to home, you may recall this line from Mason City's Meredith Willson's *Music Man* in the song "You Ought to Give Iowa a Try": *Glad to have you with us—though we may not mention it again.* And of course there are Garrison Keillor's Powdermilk Biscuits for us shy prairie people who need to *stand up and do what needs to be done.*

How did we come by our regional legacy of reserve? Partly from the national and ethnic traits of those who settled the midland: the English (with their stiff upper lips); the Scotch ("God's frozen people," according to *Omaha World Herald* columnist Robert McMorris); Scandinavians ("The Norwegian farmer loved his wife—and he almost told her" goes a well-loved joke in Decorah); the Dutch ("men of Spartan taciturnity," Washington Irving declared); those strong silent German papas, and on and on. Many Irish settled Iowa and some brought their famed "gift of the gab" with them, but Tom Kelly, who bought Kelly's Bluff in Dubuque for $300 was reputedly so reserved he would tell no one about his mine and spent his life "as uncommunicative as ever."

Beyond the national and ethnic traits of those who settled Iowa, our climate and geography have contributed greatly to our regional reserve. When it's fifty degrees below zero wind chill, we don't feel too inclined to stand around shooting the breeze on our porch swings or town squares. The isolation of our farms also encouraged the trait of silent endurance for which we are so famously known. "It could be worse," we doggedly say.

What I call "Calvinist strictness"—for better and worse—also leant a hand. We derive our much-admired Iowa work ethic from these admirable Calvinists; however, when your nose is to the grindstone, it's hard to move your lips. Grant Wood saw this and painted his famous "American Gothic" dentist and sister with both pitchfork and pinched lips.

Once you start honing in on midwestern modesty, on our culture of calm reserve, you'll start to see that across the centuries midwesterners have developed a range of strategies for dealing with our quiet culture—and I hope you'll start cultivating your own.

Writer Ernest Hemingway of Illinois made a virtue of midwestern reserve, and that's certainly one strategy: try to make the best of it. Hemingway's strong, silent-type heroes influenced several generations of Americans— and not just midwesterners. Yet these silent heroes usually were wounded and lived, when they did not die, in a climate of loss.

Tom Heggen of Mason City, the author of *Mister Roberts*, admired Hemingway, but took his very different strategy from F. Scott Fitzgerald of Minnesota. Heggen and Fitzgerald suppressed their feelings to such an extent that they split off into manic and depressive sides—both destructive. Recall flamboyant Gatsby and reserved midwesterner Nick Carraway in *The Great Gatsby* and crazy Ensign Pulver and reserved Doug Roberts in *Mister Roberts*.

Davenport playwright and novelist Susan Glaspell found a healthier strategy than either Hemingway's or Heggen's. In such world-famous works as "Trifles," about an actual 1900 Indianola murder, Glaspell makes "voicelessness" both her subject and method. The truly sensitive characters in Glaspell's works give voice and meaning to silent people's lives. Her works shout out: attention must be paid to our silent ones.

Carol Bly, the Minnesota writer, is paying attention. Bly advocates refreshing outspokenness and directness. It is no accident she wrote the foreword to *Breaking Hard Ground*, a book in which farmers give voice to their concerns and visions, or that another of her books is titled *The Passionate, Accurate Story*.

Why do I ruin your day with news of Iowa reserve? Don't we think of ourselves as among the friendliest people, always willing to lend a hand? Helping a neighbor is also part of our culture, but after the friendly hand and hello, we often find ourselves standing there tongue-tied—what to say and do next—as our deep-seated reserve kicks in.

I bother you about Iowa reserve to let you off the hook. If you've gone through life yearning for your father or your mother to say they love you, or if you wish you could be more expressive yourself of your thoughts or feelings, forgive yourself, and try to forgive them. It's not their fault, or your fault. We all labor within the midwestern climate of reserve.

Once you know you are living in a quiet culture, you can work hard to overcome its drawbacks. Modesty generally is attractive; however, too much modesty can keep you from stretching yourself, from daring to be great, from developing your gifts to their fullest potential. Hiding your light keeps us all in darkness. Once we recognize our historical legacy of reserve, Iowans must work especially hard to draw each other out—to ask questions of each other, to create more occasions for talk, to encourage daring and innovation and the hardy egos that go with them.

We don't need to give up all the things we like about ourselves as Iowans—our love of plain speech, our calm, our strong work ethic—in order to help each other be more expressive. It's not a matter of either/or—but both/and. We can work *smarter* if we talk to each other more. Most of us long to be more joyful, more expressive of a full range of thoughts and emotions. You can help yourself—and help your state in the process—by doing just that: by being more daring and expressive.

A Kalona farmer reminded me of the old saying, "The nail that sticks out gets hit." Let's rework this in the new millennium to: "The nail that sticks out gets a laurel wreath."

Sincerely,

Barbara Lounsberry

Bonnie Mansfield

Bonnie Mansfield was born on a farm in Iowa, and began her education in a one-room rural schoolhouse. Mansfield remembers vividly her farm upbringing, a lifestyle which included the wonders of hog-butchering, lard-rendering, bologna-stuffing, soap-making, and hay-stacking. After completing her education at the University of Northern Iowa, she began a teaching career, a passion that would lead to a position as educational consultant for Area Education Agency (AEA) 13 in southwest Iowa. Now retired, Mansfield enjoys volunteering in church, school, and community and staying in touch with her daughter, a nurse, and her son, a pilot for United Airlines. She describes her five grandchildren as great joys.

Dear Young Iowan:

As you look out your window and see the Rocky Mountains, what part of Iowa will you remember? What blessings and challenges? The fact that we didn't even have a stoplight in our town, and yet we could be at a Wal-Mart in thirty minutes? And when your teeth braces broke on Saturday afternoon and we called the dentist at home, he met us at the office within an hour?

Remember when your Mom would drop you off at my house before school so you could walk across the street to the elementary building? I would already have left for my classroom, but I would leave you a note. And we ended up writing notes back and forth all week. I still have those notes.

Who could forget the ceremony of freezing sweet corn, of picking gunny sacks full of golden ears, and the assembly line of husking, silking, and cutting it from the cob to hurry it into the freezer?

Perhaps one of your blessings was that you always had a car to drive, and yet your driveway was always muddy. It sometimes proved a challenge to keep between the ditches.

And how about 4-H; the challenges of getting everything ready for county fair, especially the record book? And the excitement of participating in the fair queen pageant!

After high school graduation, when you were accepted in the radiology program, we were all so proud of you, especially your mom. As a nurse, she understands what you've been through and just how important good healthcare is.

Even after you left us, you were so loyal to touch base with all the family— keeping us posted on your challenges and your hospital experiences. When you completed your certification and applied in Colorado, it was confirmation that you had a solid foundation and that you were ready for the professional world.

As I compare your growing up years in Iowa with mine, it is obvious that all your education, especially the technology you have mastered, puts you generations ahead. My farm home on a country road had no electricity or telephone during my preschool years; you have three TV sets, a DVD player, a computer, and an iPod, plus satellite in your four-wheel-drive automobile.

It was so exciting when we Iowans all converged on Colorado last month to celebrate your twenty-first birthday. We are so proud of you. As a twenty-first-century pioneer, you are blazing trails and pursuing goals. And even though you no longer claim an Iowa address, you can be sure that we will always claim you.

Keep on keepin' on,

Gram Bonnie

Renee Mauser

Sister Renee Mauser of The Redemptive Heart is foundress of Les Thereseans, a Lay Apostolate in honor of The Little Flower, Saint Therese of Lisieux, France. Les Thereseans are tertiaries, men and women who follow the Little Way and spend their day in prayer and contemplation while fulfilling missions in their personal lives out in the world.

In her letter below, Sister Renee writes to Iowan Father Louis Greving, who carried on the work begun in 1912 by Father Paul Dobberstein on West Bend, Iowa's Grotto of the Redemption. As a child, Paul Dobberstein had been gravely ill, and, according to the story, vowed that if he recovered he would build a shrine to the Virgin Mary. The result was West Bend's Grotto of Redemption and the adjacent St. Peter and Paul's Church—the product of forty-two years of Father Dobberstein's miraculous work with concrete, ornamental rocks, and semiprecious stones from around the world. Sister Renee and her order continue to take an active interest in both the church and the grotto, which receive more than 40,000 visitors a year. The Grotto is owned by the Diocese of Sioux City.

Dear Father Louis Greving:

I remember in times past the many ways you had touched my life and the lives of many others.

Your work at the Grotto of Redemption in West Bend, Iowa was a mission sent by God, and I thank you for being there for me as I answered God's call to found a new Third Order in honor of Saint Therese, The Little Flower.

I can honestly say that you and the builder of the Grotto, Father Paul Dobberstein, have enkindled a spark many times and that spark has lighted the way for much inspiration to those who may have faltered on their own. Your heavenly inspiration exceeds the tens of thousands of visitors that come to the Grotto each year and outshines the shrine's minerals and semiprecious stones, believed to be the greatest concentration of their kind anywhere in the world!

Remember when a speaker from Australia came to Stacyville, Iowa, years ago? I called several priests in the area to assist with the mission, and tried desperately to find you. You were gone, out on the road somewhere in your little camper. Your secretary did not have the means to contact you.

Yet, when I arrived early that morning to prepare for the day's activities at the Church of The Visitation, there was a very unusual, but wonderful sight!

There, in the parking lot of the church, was a very big car. Behind it sat a little silver camper! As I approached in curiosity, out stepped a priest! Yes, there you were, Father Greving, as you announced that you had been there all night, praying for the success of the mission. And, oh, what a success it was, for hundreds of pilgrims from all over the three-state area came, and the blessings were abundant.

Thank you, Father, for one of the many miracles I experienced through your intercession!

Sister Renee of The Redemptive Heart

Bill McAnally

For the past sixteen years, Bill McAnally's students have built some of the most energy efficient homes in Iowa, and many graduates of the program he coordinates at Iowa Central Community College in Fort Dodge are now successful carpenters carrying on the tradition of quality construction in Iowa—a track record that recently earned the program the Iowa Industrial Technology Education Association Program of Excellence. A contractor for fifteen years, McAnally has earned many teaching awards as an instructor of carpentry, including a Golden Apple, and Instructor of the Year from the Iowa Community College Board of Directors Association. A regular guest on Iowa Public Radio through 2006, he has become a trusted voice for home improvement in the state.

Dear Young Iowan:

You're young and full of ideas and confusion: What am I supposed to do when I grow up?

At the end of the day you will want to leave a mark—literally—that can be studied by future generations. It may be as small as a backyard deck or as large as a customer's dream home. A simple three-rail fence or a redwood gazebo. At each cut you will smell the wood scent from a tree that will go on living in your creation. You owe it to that tree to mold or shape each piece to the best of your abilities.

As a carpenter, professional or amateur, you will enjoy the camaraderie of days spent with like-minded individuals crafting both woodwork and practical jokes. You'll have the pleasure of going to bed each night looking forward to the next day's job; that anticipation is a good sign that you have chosen a pursuit worthy of a *career*.

Every morning you will rise early with the day spreading out before you. Sure, it might be ninety-five degrees and so humid that you are already on your second shirt by noon. Or the snow might be whipping behind your glasses as you try to "button up" a house before the real storm hits. On those days, no matter how miserable the working conditions, console yourself that you're going home with good fodder for storytelling, story crafting. Each project has its own life.

I'm blessed to have carpentry in my blood. My great-great-grandfather and great-grandfather were carpenters. My grandfather was an electrician; my father was a realtor and handyman. To carry on the tradition is an honor. I love looking at the parquet flooring, the houses, and structures that were crafted by my ancestors. These creations give credence to our time here on earth.

So the next time you attend a wedding in a beautiful church, analyze the roofbeams above or the ornate trim around the stained glass windows. Wonder whether the original carpenter would approve. When you start seeing with the eyes of a craftsman, whether carpentry is your day job or not, we welcome you into our fold.

So go build that treehouse, birdhouse, picket fence or deer stand. We all have that carpenter within us. Make it your life.

Have fun,

Bill McAnally

Daniel McFarland

Daniel McFarland was born on his family's Century Farm. Schooled in Fredericksburg and later educated at the University of Iowa, he served as an Air Force navigator. A retired commander, McFarland operates a ranch raising purebred polled Herefords and buffalo. The farm offers buffalo tours, meat, and legendary hunts. At age seventy-three, he has no plans to retire.

Dear Young Iowan:

One of my great rewards has been raising a family whose deep appreciation for history has allowed us to preserve our family ground, a farm *all* of our family owns. I've done what I can to preserve this farm for generations to follow. We call it a ranch now, since the return of our buffalo, but it's still a farm—a farm whose rich black soil is the most fragrant of perfumes, a farm whose trees stand tall without fear of chainsaw. You'll always be able to watch the trees here, planted like soldiers to diminish the winter winds that whip across the prairie we have lovingly restored.

You'll come to know the "Figure 4" tree, a red oak shaped by Indians. It stands above our little creek, the same creek which runs past our animal cemetery. You'll see the stones erected for those special animals we loved and appreciated.

With the coming of each spring and the rebirth of new life, you'll learn where to search for cowslips and the ever rare lady slippers. If life should take you away from Iowa, you'll come to miss the rumble of thunder and listening to the rain while sitting on the old wooden porch bench my dad made when he was first married. You'll miss the emerald green of the lawn and shimmering white fence; the old red barn and its collection of cats and chickens. Despite its century-long history, the old barn stands tall and freshly painted. It has stood strong against the Iowa storms and still retains the smell of cows and fresh-made hay. Proudly, it has not joined the ranks of its friends who have fallen from neglect and become ghosts.

And don't forget Grandma's peonies and hollyhocks. Each season their pastel colors add so much color and cheer to this place. Last, but not least, you'll not forget the yellow rosebush. It's clung to its place in the yard for over a century, always blooming on my birthday.

I hope you'll come to know that the buffalo and mustangs that roam our farm are not just an attraction. They are there to instill in others an appreciation for a time when wild animals and Indians lived in harmony. Not confined to an Americanized feedlot, our animals live free and, in the words of one of our guests, look happy.

Our country, your country, is a marvelous and majestic place. Out here on the ranch, governments and politics seem a necessary and wasteful aggravation. Still, ours is the best governmental system yet devised.

Freedom is not cheap. For eight generations, we as a family have answered the call—always volunteers, never conscripts. Since the Revolutionary and Civil Wars, we have all served. As I write, young Daniel is being sent to the Middle East; his sister has already served a tour in Iraq; their dad has served in more countries than you know exist. My twenty years in the military were very rewarding; my brother committed to nearly thirty years.

It was with humility and great appreciation that, in 2005, our family received the first-ever Five Sullivan Brothers Award for Military Commitment. To be mentioned alongside the Sullivan Brothers is an honor beyond description.

And so, my children, young Iowans all, I offer and wish you all the best in life. Life is short. Change is inevitable. So look for good and lasting things. Take advantage of and enjoy each new day. Remember the day past can never be recovered.

My love to you,

Pa

Steve McGuire

Steve McGuire is a professor at the University of Iowa, where he teaches the popular course "What Is Storytelling For?" and, along with his student storytellers, is a favorite guest on Iowa Public Radio's Java Blend. *He is also a contemporary traditional storyteller who performs across the United States and in Mexico and Canada.*

McGuire's most recent work is included on the DVD On The American Discovery Trail: Iowa Route *and* Composing byCycle Eminent Icelandic Saga and Tremendous Earth. *His current project is* Poetics of Endurance: Composing a Thing in Itself, Now, *a storytelling performance focused on his twenty-four-hour bike ride across Iowa via gravel roads.*

Dear Young Iowan:

Images demand, and they redeem. As the years go by you will realize that your life is filled with crucial moments of storymaking.

A case in point: In August 1995 I was in Prairie Lights Books in Iowa City. My wife, Lore, was looking for books on volcanoes for her seventh grade earth science class. I was paging through a book on bicycling when I came across a photograph of a man on his bike in what appeared, from his attire, to be extreme winter conditions. The caption under the photograph explained: "The Idita-bike, already half the participants have pulled out from frostbite and hypothermia. Billed as the 'world's toughest human powered ultra-marathon' the race takes place annually on the Iditarod Trail in the Alaskan bush where temperatures frequently reach forty below zero."

I took the book over to my wife and said, "Look at this, Lore!"

After she read the caption, she said, "Don't think about it, because it is not going to happen!"

Wouldn't you know, some months later, February 19, I found myself on my back at three o'clock in the morning. The thermometer on my jacket read thirty-five below zero. Location: The Iditarod Trail, Alaska.

I real quickly got my wits about me and slipped my foot back into my boot, recovering from a moment of stupidity. I'd taken my foot out because the tops of my toes had been rubbed raw from the ridge on my sock liners.

Every step I took was painful. And I'd taken a lot of steps because I'd pushed my bike the past nineteen miles. I had pushed my bike because the trail was moose-rutted—chewed up from the hooves of moose using the trail in late winter to better negotiate deep snow in the Alaskan bush—and impossible to pedal on.

As I lay on my back I asked myself, *What was I thinking when I saw that photograph?* Above, the Northern Lights cascaded green like a waterfall. And I thought, *Isn't that a magnificent image? Isn't that an image that's demanding?*

I stood up and began to gather the Nutty-Butty bars that had spilled from the bag on my handlebars, as I leaned my bike over to take off my boot. I'd bought forty-seven boxes for this race. I noticed, then, a light off in the distance approaching. Instantly it was upon me and swallowed me up—so bright and intense I had to cover my eyes and look down. And then I heard a voice. And the voice said, "Are your feet cold? Are your hands warm? Have you had enough to eat? How often do you have something to drink?"

I had been asking myself these very same questions the past three miles since coming upon a man standing in the trail, his feet so cold he could not step forward, and his hands too numb to turn the dial on his stove.

Click. The light went off. In front of me a cloud of breath hovered four feet above the ground and trailed nearly twenty feet back, at the end of which stood a kind of hero—Martin Buser. Martin Buser had, at that time, already won the Iditarod Sled Dog Race two times. He's since won it again. He looked at me and said, "You should make it to Skwentna by sun up. Good luck." And he left.

I made it to Skwentna by sun up and ate moose stew and reindeer sausage at the checkpoint. My mind was rolling on its own, so I pedaled on down the trail. Twenty hours later, fifty-one hours after the race began, I stood at the finish line. They took my photograph.

When I showed my father that photograph he asked me "What were you thinking at that moment?" I replied, "Do you remember the summer I painted a picture of my Demon Hot Wheel?" He said, "No." But he did remember when I got a job selling Cokes at the dragstrip. I told him when the camera flashed I remembered those Cokes.

A long time ago I learned a lesson about doing things that are beautiful telling. Pay attention to the pictures in your head and try to accomplish those images, and you will always be headed in the right direction.

Imagination makes and remakes you.

Yours in pictures,

Steve

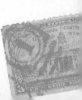

Karen Menz

A veteran schoolteacher with more than thirty years experience, Mrs. Menz, as her students know her, writes that her history students always assume she was alive in the bygone eras covered in their textbooks. She has three sons, including one, she says, who claims that her writing sounds like a third grade teacher. Menz grew up in three small Iowa towns: Cumberland (from ages 7-10), Leon (from ages 11-15), and Perry during her high school years. She counts her children lucky that they were able to grow up on an Iowa farm. Karen Menz lives and teaches in Perry.

Dear Young Iowan:

Your baseball scores were in the paper yesterday, and you were so excited to bring a copy of the newspaper into the classroom to share that your team had won. I was excited to see you so excited! You good-naturedly celebrated the other team's loss: I say good-naturedly because some of the losing team members are your classmates and your win was their loss.

The newspaper you brought sparked a memory in my mind. That newspaper appears on your doorstep or in your mailbox and I am sure you never even think about how it gets there. When I was growing up in Iowa, it got there because I put it there. I was a papergirl!

I was seven years old when I first started delivering the *Omaha World Herald* and the *Atlantic News Telegraph* in the small town of Cumberland, Iowa. Today, no one would think of sending a seven-year-old girl out on her own at 6:00 AM in the dead of winter, but in 1959 it was an opportunity in my community that I seized. It was a glorious freedom and a guaranteed source of income.

My brother Kent and I took the route together, and like all big brothers, he decided which part of the route I covered. Mine was the hilly, eastern part of town and the route actually went out into the country for quite a ways. It only now occurs to me that he chose the better route! We picked up the newspapers at the post office where they had been dropped off in bundles. We would open the bundles and then put the papers into heavy canvas bags we carried on our shoulders. And you thought your bookbags were heavy!

I remember how cold it was, especially on the morning route. Today, the weatherman tells us the "wind-chill" and you bundle up in heavy snowpants, parkas, and heavy boots. Rubber overshoes were our staple for rain or snow in those days, and I can still remember the feel of those rubber boots rubbing back and forth on my bare calves as I walked. Sometimes my legs were more chapped than my lips.

On the Sunday morning route, when the papers were especially heavy, some of my customers would show sympathy and invite me in to rest or warm up with hot chocolate. I wonder now if I would let my children go into the homes of people I don't know, and I am sure your parents caution you against ever doing such a thing. Somehow, back then, it was alright. In fact, when your fingers were frozen and your back was aching, it was more than alright.

Sometimes, too, my nostrils would stick together, frozen for just a moment, and the coal smell was stuck there all morning.

Each of my customers had a preference for where I put their paper. The newspaper would go on the porch, in the door, or sometimes clamped behind a spoon-like device nailed to the house. The cool thing about the spoon was that the bowl part held the money that paid for the paper. Today our town's newspaper costs seventy cents for each paper. The daily paper that I delivered cost twenty-five cents a week. I remember the quarter part because one customer left a half-dollar, and I was so intent on making the correct change I forgot to leave his paper!

Today your parents send their subscription fee directly to the newspaper and the carrier never touches the money. It was our job then to collect the money from each customer, send the newspaper its share, and keep the rest. To send the money to the newspaper company, though, my brother and I had to figure out how much we owed based on how many papers we were sent, buy a money order at the post office (because of course we didn't have a checking account and you couldn't send cash in the mail), and send a money order to Atlantic or Omaha.

Can you see why I am so insistent that you learn your math facts?

Besides great exercise, daily math practice, and a steady income, having a paper route had another great benefit. At Christmas my bag would be filled at the end of the route—with presents! Almost every customer had a gift for me. Now we leave the paper carrier a gift card or money in an envelope, but a real present wrapped in Christmas paper was the standard back then. My customers would sometimes leave the present on the porch, but more often they would be waiting to give it to me in person. I remember one customer so clearly, old Phenas Eblen, who lived in a tiny house and who I assumed was poor, but every Christmas there was a big bag of wavy ribbon candy for me. (He was one of my "come in and warm up" customers!)

Today I am your schoolteacher, and among the lessons I have to teach you are the lessons I wish I could teach you: to be kind to your friends, to be active, and to seize the opportunities your small town offers.

Today you showed me that you have already learned those things.

With love,

Mrs. Menz

Good Sense from the Good Folks of Iowa

Cornelia F. Mutel

Connie Mutel has lived in an oak-hickory woodland north of Iowa City since shortly after coming to Iowa in 1975. Always fascinated with Iowa's natural features and its people, Mutel and her husband have raised three sons on their land, and now welcome their young grandchildren to the woods.

Mutel, an active member in a number of natural area preservation and restoration efforts, writes frequently on natural history, an interest which has inspired her books Fragile Giants: A Natural History of the Loess Hills *and* The Tallgrass Restoration Handbook. *In her employment at the University of Iowa's IIHR—Hydroscience & Engineering, she tends archives and writes about engineering history and global change.*

Dear Young Iowan:

A few days ago, you and I took a walk in the woods near the house where your papa grew up, and where he brought you to introduce you to your grandpa and me and to your new home: Iowa—a land of grasses, once vast tallgrass prairies and oak savannas, now agricultural grasses and denser forests. For the past three years, you have come to this house every week to visit your grandpa and me. Do you know how precious those times are to me, your Oma, how much I love to hear you jump from the car and run down the gravel path to the house, clomp across the porch, open the door, and call to us? Do you realize how precious you are to me, my first and only granddaughter, my little girl who is learning to love this house of ours in the woods, and the trees and birds and bugs and chipmunks who also visit us here?

My spunky little one, my girl who knows what she wants and sets out to get it, you live with passion and energy and determination. I watch you and wonder what you will be like in ten years, in twenty, and what the world we inhabit will be like then. Life is likely to get a lot more difficult during your lifetime, as the number of people on our planet continues to grow, and as natural places like our Iowa woodlands are compressed into smaller and smaller spaces. What can I do to make sure that you and your children and grandchildren have woods and fields to explore when you grow up? What can *you* do?

I love to walk with you in our woods. I need to be patient when I do this, because it's a slow process. Very slow. The tiniest green sprout peeking from the soil needs to be stopped and examined. Each new spring wildflower needs to be discussed—why is it a certain color; why is it growing here; what shape are the leaves? We come to a log and you start to crawl over it. You stop and stare. And stare, and stare, not moving. I wait, breathe deeply, and tell myself to relax. "It's a red spider," you finally whisper, and point into a crevice in the soil where the tiny arachnid is creeping through the duff. Then you notice a patch of mushrooms under the log and we squat to rub them, smell them, pick them like flowers. On each walk, we check the progress of the deer rotting near the creek, watch how its bones are gradually being exposed and whitened, and then we talk about how endings and new beginnings circle into oneness. Our walks are deliberate processes because you see the miracle and uniqueness of each bit of natural life and insist on celebrating and exploring that miracle. You refuse to be hurried. You see what most of us miss in our hustle.

I think of your ardor, your stubbornness, your fierce love. Your spirit that leads to shrieks and stomps and that sometimes confounds your parents. I treasure your spirit's intensity. I think the world needs more like you, people who truly care. But only if that spirit is trained to care about others, and care for them—only if that spirit is focused beyond your own desires for gratification.

I watch the moths flitting around the screens at night, hear the tree frogs singing, and think how much they need you, too. And so here is my hope for you, my blond-haired treasure: that you take your passion and your lust for life, and focus it on fighting for the lives of others—the owls whose calls widen your eyes with amazement, the snakes that both frighten and fascinate you. That you shape your voice into shouts and demands for justice for the natural world and all that inhabits it. That you fight for the survival of what you are getting to know and love—just as your papa is now doing about the things he came to love when he was a boy.

Here in Iowa, just like all other intensively farmed states, you will have plenty of chances to do this. You will, as you grow, learn more about the pain of the natural world and its losses. About how the diverse prairies that once covered our state have been reduced to expanses of corn and soybeans, and about how remaining oak woodlands like ours are slowly fading from the landscape. Your parents and I will help you also learn about the natural world's possibilities. I hope that you focus on the latter and that you continue to cherish the tidbits of wildness around you, amidst Iowa's croplands and villages. I hope that you see the wildness as a window both to the creation and to your Creator, and as a door through which to release your spirit. You know the raccoons that crawl onto our deck in the night, the toads that leap and the bats that flit? They will need you to defend them, to cherish and care for them. And you will need them for your own expression, for your own wholeness.

That's both my hope and my blessing for you—that you live fully, richly, with zeal, never forgetting the meek of the earth, never forgetting your connections to all of life, never forgetting that your voice is a powerful tool to use for good. Go for it, my dear granddaughter—and world, watch out, here she comes!

Love,

Your Oma

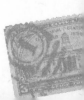

Neil Nakadate

Born in Indiana, raised in Oregon, and schooled at Stanford and at Indiana University, Dr. Neil Nakadate traveled widely before settling in Ames, Iowa. His publications have appeared in Aethlon, Cottonwood, Flyway, ISLE, Mississippi Quarterly, Western Humanities Review, Genre, Tennessee Studies in Literature, Annals of Internal Medicine, *and elsewhere, and he has edited two books on Robert Penn Warren and written a critical study of Jane Smiley's fiction. Since 1977, Nakadate has taught American literature at Iowa State University. Raised in Ames, his adult children now live and work in Houston, San Francisco, and New York.*

Dear Young Iowan:

You might try leaving. Iowa, that is. Leave. Take off.

You probably won't get this advice from most other long-time Iowans, especially if they consider you imaginative, talented, and smart. There's a lot of concern in Iowa lately about the talent drain. But still, as a frustrated parent is said to have blurted once, "If you want to go, go; if you want to stay, *go.*"

I know that sounds contrary, or even perverse, but if you've already reached adolescence and haven't discovered "contrary," then you haven't lived. And as for the attraction of places that are not Iowa, you don't need me to let you know what is out there. All that technology bombarding your eyes and ears won't let you forget that there are other songs to sing and other ways to live, in far away places with strange sounding names—nothing like *Dubuque, Clarinda,* or *Allamakee.* (This lure of the exotic has been around for centuries, by the way, since the invention of travel books or, if you prefer, since the earliest movies made available to every town with a "picture show" their adventure and "travelogue" visions of the rest of the world.)

Think of it this way: You will be adding to their diversity—the people who have never seen bacon on the hoof or soybeans by the acre, the people who have never been to a state fair or a wrestling meet, or detasseled.

Of course, you could stick around, never crossing the Missouri or Mississippi for more than a vacation, and you might even go so far as to

Good Sense from the Good Folks of Iowa

reconfirm that everything is up to date in Kansas City, but that's so … well, twentieth-century. Everything is global now—both the environmentalists and the economists tell us that the earth is the greatest show on earth—so if you really are talented and smart, consider what you might accomplish out there, where everything is different. Even a little imagination will enable you to see that "out there" is an important version of "outside the box."

By the way, once you leave, others will label you "born in," "formerly of," or "originally from," and that will grant you a certain kind of authority regarding Iowa. Curious people might even listen. But that won't mean you truly understand Iowa, or understand what you've come to love about it. I think you'll discover that just being from a particular place has only tempted you to take it for granted.

So I'll bet you'll eventually consider coming back: You'll wake up some morning in Manhattan or L.A. and realize that you forgot what it's like to sleep with the windows open. You'll realize you haven't heard crickets in a while or the insect-laden hum of a farm pond in July, or seen true winter blowing in from Nebraska or the reassuring symmetry of undulating, corn-rowed land—and you'll want to come home. At least long enough to savor spring with some rhubarb pie and to cradle tomatoes growing on a vine and not stuffed in a box.

And maybe you'll decide to stick around for a while, show off your outsider's knowledge and sophisticated skills, and give Iowa the benefit of some of the things that it hasn't been but might still become.

As I said, you might try leaving.

Sincerely,

Neil Nakadate

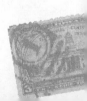

Marvin Negley

The president of the Glenn Miller Birthplace Society, an organization with fourteen hundred members around the world and a branch in Tokyo, Japan, Marvin Negley's passion for music and education have reached well beyond the southwest Iowa farm he grew up on during the 1940s and 50s. In 1991, Negley started a student exchange between Clarinda High School and Tamana Girls High School in Japan and continues to coordinate the exchange program he began.

A 1962 graduate from Iowa State University in electrical engineering, Negley comes from a technologically gifted family who have all earned degrees from ISU—his wife in mathematics and his three sons in computer engineering. Negley himself worked six years in acoustics for Electro-Voice in Michigan and then as manager of development and engineering at Lisle Corporation in Clarinda until his retirement. He and his wife have two grandsons.

Dear Glenn Miller:

When I was growing up as an Iowa farm boy, I enjoyed listening to your music. It was the Big Band era, and an unusual time in musical history, when every generation loved the same music.

I was born in 1937, the year that you started your first band. When I was seven years old in 1944, you disappeared during a World War II flight from England to France. Over the years I searched for you in your music, and I am writing to tell you why, as an Iowan, I am very proud of what you accomplished in the forty years in which you lived. I think every Iowan should be proud of you, and there are many reasons why. It is best to start from every Iowan's roots: their family.

Young Iowans today will be interested to learn that your family spent around thirty-six years in Iowa before they left Clarinda, where you were born in 1904, and from where you moved, finally, to Fort Morgan, Colorado, where you graduated from high school. In your high school years, you fell in love with a new kind of music called "dance band music" the way young Iowans today gravitate to what's popular in the dance clubs. Your interest in this music started you playing trombone with some local bands. When you graduated you skipped the ceremonies to gig with a band in Laramie,

Wyoming. Back in Fort Morgan your mother had to pick up your diploma from the high school principal, who commented, "Maybe you're the one who should get it anyway, you probably worked harder on it than he did!"

After high school, and a short taste of university life (couldn't hold your interest), you, like so many young Iowans then as now, headed for California where you got your first big break playing and arranging for Ben Pollack's Band, which led you to Chicago and a room with an up-and-coming musician and clarinet player who was to become a lifelong friend, Benny Goodman. Eventually, the Pollack band got an opportunity to play on the East Coast, and you all headed for New York City, another dream in the making.

In 1937, you decided to fulfill your grand plan of organizing your own band, but it didn't succeed financially. Not being one to give up, you tried again in 1938. This time was different, and, in March of 1939, your band was chosen to play the summer season at the prestigious Glen Island Casino, in New Rochelle, New York and at the Meadowbrook in New Jersey. Those ballrooms got you on the radio, and the audiences followed.

In the fall of 1939, you began a series of radio broadcasts for Chesterfield cigarettes which increased your popularity. Thereafter, the band was in constant demand for recording sessions and appeared in two films: *Sun Valley Serenade* in 1941 and *Orchestra Wives* in 1942. The first film included your hit song, "Chattanooga Choo-Choo" which sold over one million records, a feat for which RCA Victor awarded you a Gold Record. Later the Recording Industry Association of America picked up the idea and awarded official gold records to artists who sold a million copies of a recording, a practice that continues to this day. More trailblazing for the kid from Clarinda.

In 1942, at the peak of your civilian career when you had more hit recordings in one year than anyone before or after in the recording industry, you decided you could better serve those in uniform by enlisting yourself and, in so doing, giving up a $20,000 weekly income. Too old to be drafted at age thirty-eight, you first volunteered for the Navy but were told that they didn't need your services. Undaunted, you wrote to the Army's Brigadier General Charles Young on August 12, 1942. You persuaded the Army to accept you because, in your own words, you could "put a little more spring into the feet of our marching men and a little more joy into their hearts" via a modernized Army band. After being accepted in the Army, your civilian band played its last concert in Passaic, New Jersey on September 27, 1942. It was such a sad event that the band couldn't finish playing your theme song, *"Moonlight Serenade."*

In the Army Specialists Corps you earned the rank of captain. For the next year and a half, in addition to arranging music, you created and directed your own fifty-member band. Your goal was to build morale, to bring a touch of home to the troops, and to modernize military music. You were a talented fundraiser, and you raised millions in war bond drives all while attracting plenty of Air Corps recruits through your *I Sustain the Wings* weekly radio broadcasts.

Arriving in London, your Glenn Miller Army Air Force Band was quartered at 25 Sloane Street, an area constantly barraged by German V-1 buzz bombs. As fate would have it, you made arrangements for the unit to move to new quarters in Bedford, England. The band moved on July 2, 1944, and the very next day a buzz bomb landed in front of your old quarters, destroying the building and killing one hundred people. You had cheated fate, or so it seemed.

On December 15, 1944, you boarded a single engine UC-64A Norseman aircraft to travel to Paris, where you were to make arrangements for a Christmas broadcast. Tragically, the plane never reached France. It was never found. Without you, the band performed the scheduled Christmas concert under the direction of Jerry Gray and continued to perform even after the war ended. One of the concerts on July 1, 1945 at Nuremburg Stadium in Germany, drew a crowd of forty thousand.

Your band arrived back in the States on August 12, 1945 and played their last concert on November 13, 1945 at a National Press Club dinner in Washington, D.C., where President Harry S Truman led the crowd in a standing ovation during the opening number, "Moonlight Serenade." After the concert, Generals Dwight Eisenhower and Hap Arnold thanked the band for a job well-done and your legendary band was discharged.

The contribution by your band can best be summed up by the words of General James H. Doolittle who said, "Next to a letter from home,

Captain Miller, your organization is the greatest morale builder in the ETO [European Theater of Operations]."

I am writing you this letter now because you were as real and as personable as a letter from home to so many. And I write to let you know, wherever you are, that your family home in Iowa has been restored to its original condition circa 1904; your fans in Iowa have seen to that.

In closing, I'll refer to you by your final rank in the U.S. Army Air Corps, Major Glenn Miller. Major, you are remembered for many things: your musical style, showmanship, hard work, perseverance, and much more. But your patriotism in giving up your number-one civilian band to enlist in the United States Army Air Corps, your pioneering efforts to modernize military bands, and your supreme sacrifice for your country have caused you to be remembered as America's favorite musical patriot.

And you will always be our favorite here in Iowa.

Adios,

Marvin Negley

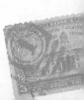

Jim Pease

Jim Pease was born in Burlington and spent much of his childhood exploring the woods and rivers near home, on foot and by canoe with his brothers. That early education led to a lifetime of wild experiences in Iowa, in the region, and internationally. Higher education took Pease to Wisconsin and Alberta, Canada, where he lived with his family in a bush cabin, studying snowshoe hares and weasels.

Since returning to Iowa in 1980, Pease has continued to spread his love of the outdoors through wilderness trips for youth and adults, through his work as Iowa State University faculty and extension wildlife specialist, and through leading international trips for students to many wild areas in the tropics. His love for wild things can be seen in the many presentations he gives around the state, including regular appearances on Iowa Public Radio. Jim and his wife, Cindy, have four grandchildren with whom they love to explore the wild.

Dear Young Iowan:

As I write this, I am sitting on a basalt rock that juts out into Lake Insula in the Boundary Waters Canoe Area Wilderness (BWCAW). The early morning fog is dancing over the lake as the sun burns through it. A mother merganser softly clucks her morning thoughts in the marsh nearby. I swat a mosquito.

Your grandma and I are on this trip with a couple of friends, one a Brazilian woman whom we are introducing to the American wilderness for her first time. Her reactions are similar to yours the first time I brought you here two summers ago. Your laughter and joy and amazement will stay with me forever and inspire me to bring your brother and cousins here, too, in the years to come. As you know, the BWCAW is one of my favorite wild places in the world, and I've been fortunate enough to see quite a few.

That brings me to the first point of this letter: I bring you here, as I did your father before you, so that you will know what wildness is. We don't have "big" wildness in Iowa any more, those areas of thousands or hundreds of thousands of acres that are "untrammeled" by humans. That means there are no roads or buildings or other things that we do to "civilize" the wild.

We are just visitors here, altering it as little as possible in our visits. As a result, the lakes are clean and wonderfully swimmable, the fish are many and wonderfully fishable, and the wild views are everywhere, wonderfully watchable. And the mosquitoes are here too, by the bizillions, unsprayed and uncontrolled. They keep us humble and remind us that we are but one of the many thousands of species with whom we share the Earth. They bug lots of other critters, as well. I'm sure they drive wolves and moose and lynx and rabbits crazy, too, just like us!

Oh, yeah, that first point: wildness is important in human lives, so I want you to know it firsthand. Soak in all you can while you can. Get out there and run and play in it—build forts, camp, fish, swim, hunt, canoe, and hike. Drink it deeply and be awed and amazed and humored and humbled by it. It will keep you in contact with your wild side.

But don't just drink in the "big" wild—those important "official" wild areas designated by The Wilderness Act. Iowa still has lots of wildness, even though the big wild was long ago tamed. We are rich in streams and rivers, prairies and woods. We have county and state parks, wildlife refuges and state preserves, big reservoirs and small ponds, restored wetlands and reconstructed prairies. Get out and explore those. After all, they are what we've left behind for you, part of your natural heritage. I've slapped my share of mosquitoes in those areas, too.

It's not a lot, to be sure. Iowa ranks next-to-last in the nation in the percentage of land that is publicly owned. Only about two percent of our land is owned by and for the public at large. That's not much, but many of the pieces are very high quality. I hope you'll take in and experience wildness whatever its size. It's good for your spirit.

That leads me to my second point: don't be complacent. Wild areas, big or small, are under constant threat. Not everyone thinks as we do. Many people, perhaps not wanting to acknowledge their wild side, don't like wildness. They want to tame and "civilize" it all, turn it into mowed parks, filled with nice roads and neat flowerbeds and benches. Some want to make the wild into the fake wild: golf courses with manicured greens and tamed "roughs" and artificial sand and water traps, all carefully planned to challenge the golfer. The "weeds" (wild plants) are herbicided; the "pests" (wild insects) are insecticided. Even the Canada geese that have decided they like the abundant grass and available water are managed so that golf shoes don't step in too much goose poop. Other folks want to turn wild areas into theme parks. They can then create "wild" experiences, complete with exciting rides, holograms of creatures, and maybe even some real live critters performing "tricks" taught them by their human trainers.

Don't get me wrong: manicured parks, golf courses, and theme parks all have their place, but it's definitely *not* in the few truly wild places we have left. The challenges and excitement and beauty that all these carefully managed places promise are there in abundance in the real wild already.

So don't take the wild for granted. Be vigilant. Get involved. Get your friends involved. Attend hearings. Join with other like-minded people in conservation organizations. Speak up. Contact your legislators at the Statehouse and in Congress and let them know how you feel. The wild places we have didn't happen by chance. People before us spoke up and got organized and convinced their elected representatives to vote to make these wild areas "permanent." But, in a democracy, their permanence can be changed. I believe we owe it to those people who worked so hard to establish them to make sure our wild areas remain wild. And we owe it to the many other wild critters that live in those wild places and have no voices in our legislatures. We, you and I, must raise our voices for them, too—even for the mosquitoes I've slapped while writing this!

Every time I'm out in the wild, I see things I've never seen before. Perhaps my eyes were not focused enough, or my mind was distracted, or maybe I didn't know how to see. As I get older and learn more, I realize how much I have left to learn. That's the thing about wild places and wild things: they have lots to teach us! You could not have convinced me, twenty years ago, that bald eagles would ever nest again in any large numbers in Iowa. The Iowa landscape, I thought, was just too tame and eagles were too wild. But the eagles taught me otherwise, and we now have nearly two hundred active eagle nests in Iowa. That is a testament to the resilience of the eagle and a testament to those folks who spoke up and got DDT banned. Clearly, as a young wildlife biologist, I had a lot to learn. Wild eagles had much to teach me.

The same is true in that little patch of prairie your grandma and I have been trying to reconstruct. We've been at it for years, planting, mowing, burning—and watching! Each year, some plant we never thought was there appears or blooms for the "first time." Was it there before? Maybe. Or maybe we just didn't see well enough. Maybe our management brought it back or maybe prairie is more resilient than we ever imagined, reappearing years after domestic cattle first grazed it. We don't yet know. Wild plants have much to teach us.

That leads me to my third point: be curious. Wild places and wild things have much to teach us but only if we are open to learning. Observe. Listen. Read. Experiment. You'll be constantly amazed at how much you have left to learn and excited at how much fun it is. I know I am.

So get out there and explore the wild. Get involved in whatever ways you can to keep the wild, and be open to learning all that the wild has to teach you. And slap a few mosquitoes for me while you're out there!

Much love,

Grandpa Jim

Sally J. Pederson

Former Lieutenant Governor Sally Pederson is a native of Vinton and a graduate of Iowa State University. She is a former executive at Meredith Corporation in Des Moines, where she was the senior food editor for Better Homes and Gardens. *She was elected Lieutenant Governor in 1998, and re-elected to a second, four-year term in 2002.*

Pederson received the 2003 John F. Sanford Award from the Iowa Medical Society in recognition of her "dedicated and tireless efforts to improve the quality of health care in Iowa." In August 2004, she was inducted into the Iowa Women's Hall of Fame. Pederson is the honorary chair of the Iowa Mentoring Partnership, dedicated to recruiting mentors and connecting Iowa children and teens with supportive adult role models. She is also the former chair of the Iowa Democratic Party.

Dear Young Iowan:

I, too, was once standing looking out on the world as a recent graduate, weighing the vast land of opportunities in front of me—ready to spread my wings for the first time, and trying to find the best place to fly. After graduating from Iowa State, I accepted a job in Des Moines and made it my home.

Our global economy now offers you countless more opportunities than were available to me. We are lucky to live in a world with so much at our fingertips. But with all of the great advances in technology and with all of our innovative American companies making headway around the globe, you will now find yourselves competing for jobs not just against other graduates from Iowa or the U.S.; instead, you will be applying for some of the same positions as young people from almost every country on the planet.

Your generation and the ones to follow will live and work in a world that is completely interconnected. You will need to have a strong foundation to compete with your peers around the globe. This foundation comes from the computer skills, math, science, and strong verbal and written communication skills you have gained here in Iowa.

As you begin to enter the work force, some of you may choose to start your career in Iowa and to you I say congratulations; we are pleased and proud to have you stay.

Some of you, no doubt, will pursue jobs beyond our borders. To you I say good luck; we know that you will be positive ambassadors for Iowa.

By all means, explore these opportunities—travel to other places, experience other cultures, and meet and learn from many different people. All of these diverse experiences will make you a more valuable employee and citizen—besides the fun you will have along the way.

But remember this: our invitation to come back home to Iowa is an open-ended invitation to return for a few days or for a lifetime. We are proud of you and you are always welcome here.

So when you are ready to settle down and raise a family, I hope you will come to the same conclusion I did: Iowa is the best place to live, learn, work, and raise a family. When you consider access to health care, quality education, safe neighborhoods, strong communities, and job opportunities nowhere else compares to our state. Iowa ranks high in all of these areas, and that is why I choose to live here, learn here, work here, and raise my family here.

Good luck on your journeys, but remember your home.

Along the way of your journey, I offer you one piece of advice: one of the core responsibilities for those who are leaders and who have been blessed with talents is service to others. And not just service, but selfless service. Your potential isn't truly realized until you do well not only for yourself and your organizations but for those most in need of your help, those less fortunate who benefit from knowing that you care. Our society has to more completely understand the need to raise ourselves up as a whole and to lessen the divide between the haves and the have-nots.

We pride ourselves on these types of values and the ethic of selfless service here in Iowa, and I hope that the memory of this mindset is threaded in your core being.

I wish you all the best in your future endeavors. I hope that you reach for noble goals and that you achieve success.

Sally J. Pederson

Bob Peterson

A resident of Cedar Rapids, Bob Peterson has worked in the industrial technical publishing field as a technical writer and graphic artist for thirty-eight years. Peterson's varied publications range from technical articles and stories published in automotive books to a forthcoming fine art reference book to be titled European and American Painting: A Reference Guide.

With a diverse educational background that includes study in photography as well as mechanical engineering design, Peterson lists art history, fine art painting, and drawing among his interests. He has also been a productive artist, exhibiting portraits at the Dubuque Museum of Art and the Hoover Presidential Library.

Dear Young Iowan:

Ask your parents and grandparents about their experiences during tough times. Make a study of those times at the same time you cherish your freedom, as I have come to cherish mine in my sixty-three years as an Iowan.

After I graduated from high school, I had my own tough times. I knew that I was not ready to attend a two-year or four-year college, so I enlisted in the U.S. Army for three years. The time was September 1962. One month later, October 1962, the human race experienced one of its greatest crises: the Cuban Missile Crisis.

Like other Americans, I was very concerned with what the future would bring. As we now know, the world came close to destruction. In the forty-four years that have passed since that terrible period, I have never missed voting in an election. Some people may say that your vote doesn't count. Don't believe them.

Since that time, I have dedicated myself to becoming an artist; maybe you are an artist, too. Even if you're not, please consider, as you seek your place in life, learning this secret from artists: do what you really like to do and do it your own way. Over the years, for example, I've read hundreds of books on the fine arts. But I was never able to find a certain type of reference book. So in 1992 I decided to write the book I always wanted, the one that never existed. It took me over twelve years to complete.

Write your own book, too, if the book you need doesn't exist, and contemplate your life and your losses in it.

Last March I lost my mother. During the week of her funeral, I helped my father with many errands and tasks. During lunch on the last day I would be in town, I thanked him for all the things that he and my mother did for me through the years. Little did I know this would be the last time I talked to my father. He died a couple of weeks later.

Appreciate the time you spend with your family, grandparents, and friends. When you finish reading this letter, thank your parents and your grandparents for all the things they have provided.

When my parents bought their house in 1942, they planted a maple tree in their front yard. When I was a young teenager, this beautiful maple was about six inches in diameter. When its leaves changed in the fall to a bright gold, it was the most beautiful tree in all of northwest Mason City. Ten years ago my parents gave me a four feet tall sapling from their maple. I planted it in my yard and now my maple tree is six inches in diameter. It provides the same golden show every fall.

Six months after my parents' death, their golden maple started to die. Mine lives on, and one day I, too, will give a sapling, so it may live on.

Survive. Never give up on your goals. It's the people who quit who don't accomplish.

As Henry Wadsworth Longfellow once said, "If you knock long enough and loud enough at the gate, you are sure to wake somebody." I did.

Now it's your turn.

Sincerely,

R.D. (Bob) Peterson

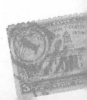

Terry Pitts

Terry Pitts has been executive director of the Cedar Rapids Museum of Art since 2000. He previously served as director and curator of the Center for Creative Photography, a museum of twentieth-century photography at the University of Arizona. He has written numerous books and articles on the history of photography—especially on the life and art of Edward Weston. Born in St. Louis and raised in the Midwest, Pitts studied at the University of Illinois, Champaign-Urbana, where he received a BA in literature and an MS in library science. He received an MA in art history from the University of Arizona. He lives in Cedar Rapids with his wife, Kathy Hall, who has taught him to love kayaking on Iowa's rivers.

In the letter to a young Iowan below, Terry Pitts imagines what Grant Wood's sister Nan might have written in a letter to her rambling brother in 1920.

A letter to Grant Wood, Summer 1920

Dear Brother:

I hope you and Marvin Cone weathered the transatlantic voyage in good spirits. Did you do any sketching on the ship? I imagine that looking out across nothing but ocean and sky for days is about as exciting as watching corn grow.

I envy your summer in Paris. Paris must seem crowded, sophisticated, and thrilling compared to Iowa. Here the humidity is settling in, the corn is rising, and everything seems—well—routine. I bought a new gramophone record that I think you'll enjoy when you get back: "How 'Ya Gonna Keep 'Em Down on the Farm? (After They've Seen Paree)." I can just see you in a French beret, spending all your time in museums and cafes!

A few days ago I had a premonition that you would never return to Cedar Rapids. But then I remembered that you've already left Iowa three times, and you've always come back to your family and friends. First you went to Minneapolis to study art right after high school. Then to Chicago for classes at the Art Institute—you scared me then because you stayed away a couple of years. Then off to join the Army for a spell.

You belong here in Iowa and I think you know it.

I think you made a great decision to concentrate more on painting after you left the Army, and I hope your time in Paris gives you a big boost in confidence. I can tell that you really enjoy tromping around the outdoors making paintings.

Because I've never been outside of the good old U.S.A. I'm depending on you—well, on your paintings—to show me what's so special about France. In fact, I send you a challenge! Try to get out of Paris one day and visit the countryside. Try to find a French version of Iowa and make a painting just for me. What do French farms look like? Do they paint their barns red like we do? Walking home from town the other day I started wondering what someone from France would think of Iowa. But you know what? It's really hard to look at something as familiar as the back of your hand—and I mean really *look*, the way an artist like you looks. I just don't have the knack! To me, a cornfield is the most monotonous thing in the universe—all those perfect rows of identical cornstalks.

You and Marvin may laugh at me, but I would think the most marvelous trick an artist could pull off would be to make an Iowa cornfield look *interesting*. As for me, I think the only way I could ever get excited about looking at a cornfield would be from the cockpit of one of the Jennys in the flying circus that came to town last week. Just imagine being three hundred feet up in the air, spooking the cows and making all the dogs bark. I'll bet Iowa looks like a patchwork quilt from up there. You should have seen them do loop-the-loops and barrel rolls! If I'd had three bucks, I could have taken an aeroplane ride myself.

I guess you can look at Iowa differently from me because you've traveled more, and I expect you'll come back with fresh eyes for Iowa. In the meantime your mother and I and all your friends say hello.

Love,

Nan

194

John Price

John Price is a writer and university professor born in Fort Dodge. He earned his BA in religion, MFA in nonfiction writing, and PhD in English at the University of Iowa, and is currently the Jefferis Chair of English at the University of Nebraska at Omaha. He is the author of numerous published essays on Iowa and the Midwest, as well as the nonfiction book, Not Just Any Land: A Personal and Literary Journey into the American Grasslands, *and was recently awarded a creative writing fellowship from the National Endowment for the Arts. He lives with his wife and two young sons in Council Bluffs.*

Dear Young Iowan:

Please stay.

Or go away and return—the sooner the better. Migration is as native to this prairie land as settlement. Think of the seasons, the birds, the once grand motion of bison and elk. This place needs you, as it does them, to be sustained and restored. To heal.

I know what you're up against, because I was up against it, too. You look around and see corn and beans and rivers and sidewalks, which can be pleasant enough, but you long for more. More grandeur. More wildness. More free, unfenced space in which to explore and get lost and find faith. You sense, even if you don't know, what is missing: a diversity of life that once rivaled the Amazonian rainforests, the great prairies and savannas and wetlands. Less than one percent of these native habitats remain, the worst record in the union. Let's not even mention the polluted water. This is what they have left you of God's creation here. And they wonder why you want to leave—for a summer, for a lifetime.

I know what you're up against, because I was up against it, too. You have talent—intellectual, physical, spiritual—and you want it to be nurtured and appreciated. You want to be around others whose talents are nurtured and appreciated. One measure of that is the public celebration and support of cultural diversity—in the arts, in education, in business, in religious belief, in human expressions of love and community. You see this diversity elsewhere, in growing places, and you want more of it here. Another measure is money and how it is shared. You know that this is an immensely wealthy country, yet you are sitting in an overcrowded classroom, next to friends whose parents (or your own) are unemployed or working several jobs, in a town selling itself to corporate "benefactors" only to be abused and abandoned by them. It's not like this for everyone—it shouldn't be—and that's part of why you wince when people talk about the Heartland. Where's the Heart?

I know what you're up against, and I still hope you'll stay. I stayed and am grateful for it—this place is worthy of the best you and I have to offer. I do not say this out of self-importance (Iowans are, in general, a humble lot) but because I believe no place should take for granted the passion and talents of its people, young or old. By staying put, the place I once wanted to escape has taught me how to see the world in a new and better way, with a degree of hope I could've hardly discovered on my own. I still feel doubt and anger—as anyone does about their home—but Iowa has taught me not to rush off from any situation without taking at least a second, more careful look. Here are just a few of the results:

Where I once saw only fences and cropland, I now see native prairie plants hanging on in the margins and in miraculous prairie preserves. They need our protection.

Where I once saw a place empty of its native wildlife, I now see the trumpeter swans and the bison and the river otters and the mountain lions returning to home ground. They need our help.

Where I once only worried about polluted waters, I now see the heroic efforts of those working to heal them. They need our encouragement.

Where I once saw only dying rural and urban communities, I now see citizens working creatively to save those communities. My definition of community has broadened to include those not only joined by common civic boundaries, but by a common vision. They need our imaginations.

Where I once wished for a place without intolerance and hate and economic injustice, I have learned to transform that longing into something tangible, through teaching and writing and raising children with moral consciences, even as I work to improve my own. Others are doing the same and we need your courage.

Where I once saw religious rigidity, I have come to understand the immense power of grace, an unearned love that can be applied to places as well as people. We need your faith.

So I know what you're up against, and I still hope you'll stay. Stay because of, and in spite of, what Iowa means to you: its brokenness and beauty, its peril and promise. You are an Iowan and that means you are willing to work when others have surrendered and fled. That is our heritage, and it is still used against us. Too often, we have lent our talents and vision to those who do not need or value them. Sometimes those people live elsewhere; sometimes they are our neighbors. That's how it will always be, but you are an Iowan and, whether you know it or not, you have learned to flourish inside conflict. Brokenness and beauty. Peril and promise. Iowa has always been a place where extremes have come together—in the sky, on the earth— and we who reside here will determine whether that coming together will ultimately be destructive or redemptive.

Stay because we need you, because this is your home and to have a home as good as this, despite its problems and imperfections, is no small thing in today's world. It is a privilege and an opportunity and, though I can't promise much, I can promise this: you will not be alone. You will be among family and friends and others, like me, who are strangers, but who are bound to you by the land we share and by the vow of all committed love: to be there, to try.

Where is the Heart in the Heartland? Beating inside your chest.

Trent D. Reedy

Trent Reedy has lived in Iowa all his life. He earned his Bachelor's degree from the University of Iowa and served in the Iowa Army National Guard. Presently, Trent teaches high school English and is pursuing a Master of Fine Arts degree. A Star Trek fan since the early nineties, he lives with his wife in Riverside, where he attends Trek Fest each year, having won first place in the Star Trek costume contest twice.

Dear Young Iowan:

Forty years ago a man named Gene Roddenberry set out to create a television show that would be both an adventurous "wagon train to the stars" and a vision of a grand future for humanity—a future that would include gender-bending characters and mind-bending races all aboard the iconic starship *Enterprise*. Since the crew of this ship was comprised of the best that a united and prosperous humanity had to offer, it was natural that the *Enterprise* would have to be commanded by an extraordinary captain from an extraordinary place.

Captain James Kirk was played by Canadian-born actor William Shatner, but by the time Star Trek made its way to the big screen in movies, it was decided that the captain of Earth's most famous future starship had to be an American. Even better, he had to be an Iowan, as we find out in the fourth Star Trek film, wherein Kirk discloses his birthplace. The fifth Star Trek movie, directed by William Shatner himself, includes still another nod toward Iowa with James Kirk's fond memories of growing up in the Hawkeye State.

Why Iowa, of all the far off places in the galaxy? Perhaps it is because of Kirk's deep sense of patriotism, as declared in his passionate speech on the virtues of freedom and the U.S. Constitution in the original series episode "The Omega Glory." Maybe Star Trek writers and producers understood the independent and self-reliant natures of the people of Iowa well enough to attribute Iowan's concern for the greater good to Captain

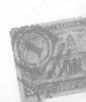

Kirk, who likewise (sometimes) violated Starfleet policy for the greater good. Whatever the reason, Captain James T. Kirk is undeniably heroic and completely Iowan, though he is, of course, fictional.

Why should young Iowans care about all of this? The answer is that a great many people are interested in Captain James T. Kirk and where he grew up. Obviously, when a show like Star Trek has spawned ten major motion pictures and four spin off television series with the total of just over seven hundred episodes, people from all around the world are interested.

Indeed, the appeal of Captain Kirk and Star Trek was sufficiently widespread to merit, in 1985, the Riverside, Iowa, city council's unanimous vote to seek permission from Star Trek creator Gene Roddenberry for recognition as the official future birthplace of the captain. Recognition granted, Riverside set up Trek Fest, a town celebration held for the past twenty-two years every last Saturday in June.

So even though Captain Kirk isn't scheduled to be born until March 22, 2233, Trekkies can still come experience some of his "heritage"—some of what made James T. Kirk the legend he will, paradoxically, become. At Trek Fest, you can watch a demolition derby, tractor pulls, and a greased pig-catching contest. You can take part in the Star Trek market and swap meet as well as a Star Trek costume contest. Star Trek movies and episodes are shown in a red barn. There's an enormous model starship, the U.S.S. Riverside, and even a life-size shuttlecraft. And, of course, you can always visit the stone monument dedicating the exact site of Captain Kirk's future birth.

At Trek Fest you will usually find people dressed up as fictional alien characters; it is also not uncommon to find real people who have traveled from faraway places on Earth—St. Louis, Boston, even Finland. That a small Iowa farm town has become internationally famous is both a tribute to the incredible influence and popularity of Star Trek, as well as an homage to the people of Iowa and the ideals they represent.

Iowans have a reputation for honesty, integrity, and a quiet unyielding strength. We are recognized for those qualities by people across the country, some of whom have rarely, if ever, set foot here. As you grow up Iowan, relish this paradoxical state—often overlooked, frequently misplaced—whose virtues have become famous around America, the world, and even around the galaxy.

Sincerely,

Trent

Rachelle H. Saltzman

Rachelle H. (Riki) Saltzman is the folklife coordinator for the Iowa Arts Council, a division of the Department of Cultural Affairs. She was born and reared in Wilmington, Delaware and has a BA in history from the University of Delaware. Her MA in history and PhD in anthropology/folklore are from the University of Texas at Austin.

Riki Saltzman came to Iowa in February of 1995 to be the curator for Iowa's portion of the Smithsonian's 1996 Festival of American Folklife in Washington D.C. and the 1996 Sesquicentennial Festival of Iowa Folklife. Saltzman is involved in place-based food research for the Leopold Center for Sustainable Agriculture and also works with a variety of Iowa folk and traditional artist groups, educators, and organizations on programming ("Cultural Express: Traditional Arts on Tour"), curriculum (Iowa Folklife: Our People, Communities, and Traditions)*, and a radio series* (Iowa Roots) *in collaboration with Iowa Public Radio.*

Dear Young Iowan:

As a non-native Iowan, I occasionally get a little peeved when the powers-that-be go on about keeping Iowans in Iowa. A good place has people from all over—from home and away.

After more than eleven years here, I am struck by the changes and the ever-widening circles and diversities of communities in Iowa—the ways in which so many people from so many places have combined their original cultures with those that have come before and from those they encountered on their journeys here. In small town and urban areas, new Iowans from Mexico, Russia, Somalia, Sierra Leone, Colombia, Guatemala, Cambodia, Vietnam, and Laos try to hold on to their heritage. As for their predecessors from France, England, Ireland, Scotland, the Germanic and Slavic states, Scandinavia, Greece, Mexico, and Italy, precious customs and keepsakes become both painful and treasured memories, as newcomers must always adapt to new environments, combine their traditions with new ones, and somehow make the transition to becoming Americans.

Iowa communities, old and new, with their eager spirit of neighborliness are our state's greatest strength. Iowans have long been generous to immigrants who long to re-establish the ties, the neighbors, and the networks they had in their homelands. From the beginning, Iowa has welcomed newcomers, a process that started in 1870 with *Iowa: A Home for Immigrants*—a booklet published by the Iowa Board of Immigration that touted the advantages of moving to Iowa from the eastern United States and from all over Europe. One hundred years later, Governor Robert Ray extended an Iowa welcome to the Tai Dam refugees from the Vietnam War. That program has grown to include people from places as far-flung as Sudan, Bosnia, and Iraq, to name only a very few.

For all the groups that have come here, their traditional foods are the nearest and dearest reminders of home, of childhood, of a safe and secure haven. For immigrants, absent foods become visceral reminders of their loss, hence the critical importance of ethnic-specific food markets and restaurants. But these enterprises not only cater to their own but also to customers from other cultural groups—curious foodies, committed sponsor families, those who have lived in other places, and, eventually, the general public. In the past decade, food markets, bakeries, and restaurants featuring Latino, Asian Indian, Southeast Asian, Russian, and Bosnian foods have multiplied throughout the state.

Eating, like listening to music or going to museums, provides a window into other cultures. We can visit places where food is grown, made, and processed—on farms, at farmers' markets, in restaurants, at festivals, in ethnic shops and bakeries. Through food, we can experience with all five of our senses—the irresistible aromas of State Fair funnel cakes and turkey legs, the crackle of popcorn popping, the seductive sight of giant Iowa cinnamon rolls lathered with thick, white icing, the succulence of giant pork tenderloins, the crisp and fluffy texture of Meskwaki fry bread. Northern and central European immigrants brought Czech red cabbage and bread dumplings, Swedish potato sausage, and Dutch pancakes to Iowa. Middle Eastern, African, Latino, and Southeast Asian immigrants have gifted us with Bosnian pita, *Nuer yot-yot* bread, Vietnamese *phở*, Mexican tamales, and Lebanese flatbread. All these foods create the "tastes" found in Iowa today.

Iowa food specialties vary somewhat by region, with smoked, fried, or pickled fish available at river cafés along the Mississippi, Missouri, and inland waterways; *flaekesteg* (pork loin embedded with prunes) and *rødkal* (red cabbage) in the Danish Inn in western Iowa (Elk Horn); *kolaches* in the east and northeast (Cedar Rapids). You can find spring rolls and savory soups at Lao, Vietnamese, and Thai restaurants in central and western Iowa (Ames, Des Moines, Sioux City, and Storm Lake); Dutch marzipan-filled pastry "letters" in Dutch settlements in southeast and northwest Iowa (Pella and Orange City); German sausages in western Iowa; and Italian sausage in Des Moines. Muscatine, Des Moines, West Liberty, and Storm Lake (all towns with significant Latino populations) produce tamales, tortillas, and pan dulces as well as feature butcher shops with razor-thin, hand-sliced beef for fajitas, cleaned tripe, *chorizo*, and *chicharones* (fried spiced pork rinds). In Tama in central Iowa, home of the Meskwaki Settlement, Indian frybread and Indian tacos are available at annual powwows and in restaurants. Visitors to northeast and north central Iowa (Decorah and Story City) can savor Norwegian treats such as *römmegrot* (a sweetened cream pudding), *lefse* (a potato flatbread), and even *lutefisk*—also available in the frozen foods section of many Iowa food markets. And locker-smoked fish and meats can be found all over the state, as can the ubiquitous and always huge fried or grilled pork tenderloin (served with mustard and pickles, of course!).

But culinary tourism, a phrase coined by Lucy Long, a folklore friend and colleague in Ohio, isn't just about visiting a new place to taste new food; it also includes really exploring and experiencing the places where food is grown, made, and processed. In Iowa, visitors and residents travel to the Amana Colonies, not just to visit the museum or buy a basket, but also to experience the past via the home-cooked, German-style meals and fresh-baked breads and pies. Those who gain entrée into the still extant Amana Church Society community can further experience rhubarb wine, potato dumplings, homemade applesauce from local apples, and what I suspect may be the prototype for that all-American green bean casserole—but the cream, string beans, and onions don't come out of a can.

Travelers to Decorah's Nordic Fest experience a variety of Norwegian foods such as *krumkake*—cream-filled butter cookies—taste locally grown organic food at town restaurants and the local food co-op; and visit the famous Decorah Hatchery. Come to the Czech and Slovak Museum and

Library in Cedar Rapids to celebrate Houby Days—in honor of those wonderful morel mushrooms that grow wild in Iowa in the early spring. Ironically, because these grow wild, they can no longer be sold in grocery stores, though you can sometimes buy them from individuals in hardware store parking lots or farmer's markets, be gifted by friends, or even hunt for your own.

In twenty-first century Iowa, foods become cultural intersections, where old and new collide. Iowa food market chains now sell both ersatz and Americanized, as well as authentic, Bosnian, Mexican, Jewish, Southern U.S., Italian, and Asian foods. Many Lao-owned food stores feature a range of foods for different Asian groups from Indian to Vietnamese. In Storm Lake and Sioux City, Asian stores also feature Mexican foods and vice versa. A foray into Des Moines Latino markets reveals *Salsa Inglesa* (Worcestershire sauce) and plastic mortars and pestles. Ethnic-specific stores tend to feature a variety of items, rather like the old general stores. Bosnian shops in Waterloo sell delectable homemade pastries and pastas, baking pans, cooking pots, and coffee paraphernalia as well as a variety of fruit syrups, coffees, and pickled vegetables. At all of these stores, customers are as likely to be waited on by checkers from the Sudan or Bosnia as from Ottumwa or Elk Horn.

Iowa today bears witness to the population and consequent cultural shifts that happen periodically in the United States. Within the past ten years, Latinos have become the largest minority group in the state, with African Americans a close second. And, clearly, not all instances of cultures coming together are positive ones. Issues of illegal immigrants, English language learning, teacher and social worker funding, and domestic relations are all potential areas of conflict. Different religious beliefs, food prohibitions, notions about time, the importance of family and community versus the pressures of the workplace, and attitudes about modern medical procedures versus traditional remedies are all issues that have been faced before. In addition to day-to-day help, newcomers also encounter prejudice, hate, and, to their ways of thinking, irrational laws and rules. Storm Lake, Marshalltown, and Postville as well as Dubuque, Des Moines, Perry, West Liberty, and Waterloo, among many Iowa towns and cities, have been targeted by outside media for their difficulties—and rarely for their successes.

These days, we fear so much—disease, contamination, pollution, difference. That fear threatens the unique tastes and places in our vast country. Fast food restaurants, sanitized amusement parks, and chains of all types make it easy to travel the landscape and never once try anything local, new, or different. We have so homogenized our food that many of us, especially young Iowans, scarcely know what it is to taste fresh, local food made from scratch. Despite a heritage of diverse family farms and strong ethnic cultures, Iowa has become better known for its agricultural commodities of corn, soybeans, hogs, and cattle than for its table food.

So here's the dilemma: do we really want people from both coasts and major urban areas to discover Iowa and all its great places, foods, and cultures? Or do we want to keep it all for Iowans?

Good places attract good people—note that Austin, Portland, Seattle, Atlanta, New York City, Madison, or Chapel Hill do not have any problem attracting residents. Interestingly, and something that few Iowans bring up, neither do Iowa City nor Decorah. I haven't noticed that Des Moines, Sioux City, or Marshalltown are losing population either. And check out Fairfield, Storm Lake, Spencer, or Cedar Rapids. All are thriving and increasingly diverse and livable places to work, buy a home, raise a family, buy and eat good food, and get involved with the community.

Photographs © Ed Heffron

Myrna Sandvik

Myrna Sandvik grew up on a traditional family farm near Lake City. For much of her adult life she taught English, speech, and French in high schools in and around Cedar Falls. Later, she tried her hand at teaching college-aged students at Hawkeye Community College and at the University of Northern Iowa, where she was an editorial assistant for the North American Review. *Currently, she teaches adult creative writing at the Hearst Center for the Arts in Cedar Falls.*

Sandvik has earned BA, MAE and MA degrees, all from UNI. A writer as well as a teacher and occasional editor, she has had several poems published in the Iowa Poetry Association annual Lyrical Iowa *as well as a collection of poetry entitled* RFD Iowa. *Sandvik has three grown children—Ron, Loren, and Katrina—and three grandchildren—Kyri, Carson, and Colton. She lives with her husband, Leonard, on a small acreage near Brandon, Iowa, where she writes and gardens.*

Dear Young Iowan:

You are lucky enough to be a member of the Hawkeye State. That membership comes with certain expectations. I will try to give you a few clues.

There is not really a fraternity handshake, but a certain talent for watching your feet intently as your toes dig arcs in the dust and your heels dig solid little holes inside those same arcs during conversation seems to be native to real Iowans. You can vary the pattern as you gain mastery, but this basic procedure will get you by. The skill that must be learned to accompany this ritual is to properly mumble unintelligible replies to any difficult question in such a way as to sound too ignorant for the questioner to believe there could be any gain from continuing the inquisition. This is important multitasking to accomplish if you wish to seem authentic to older Iowans.

It will also be necessary for you to learn long-distance spitting. One fine point of that is checking the wind direction before the first salvo. This is an important skill because an experienced Iowa spitter conveys most of the emotional content of conversations, especially negotiations, with the distance and timing of spit shots.

For example, if there is a great hacking sound before the missile flies, usually missing the other conversant's shoe by less than a hair's breadth, the mood is contempt. If the spittle floats quietly off to the outside of the conversational circle, you are dealing with chagrin, sometimes called "the gotcha" in other cultures. Finally there is the "leave me alone, I'm thinking" message which usually is just quiet and continuous small gobs landing not too far from the spitter's own feet.

This entire series must be completed without ever making eye contact with anyone else during the whole procedure. The minute you look up to see if anyone is impressed, the spell is broken, and it is time to confess what thoughts have absorbed so much of your attention.

A good technique here is to have a decent thought planned ahead if you really want to think about something that really is private, like: whether the new girl in class noticed you yesterday when you cannonballed off the diving board and splashed water all over her. It would not be cool to admit anything so private. One good cover, "I don't think it will rain tonight," always works unless, of course, it is already storming. You are smart. You can think of other good distractions, now that you know the basic rules.

The last essential thing for you to know is that you must learn to be obsessed with the weather. That is the real trademark of a true Iowan. In other states the weather is a fleeting thing passing almost unnoticed. In Iowa the weather is more important than *what's for dinner?* You can be right or wrong. You can like heat or cold. You can be optimistic or pessimistic. But you cannot be indifferent. You must take a position and defend it passionately and listen just as passionately to everyone else's position.

A simple rule of thumb is that, in Iowa, the weather occupies the same importance as film stars always have in Hollywood.

With these few simple rules, I leave you on your own to navigate the special pitfalls of the Iowa social scene.

Sincerely,

Myrna Sandvik

Ron Sandvik

Ron Sandvik is the managing editor of the North American Review *at the University of Northern Iowa. He has jumped off shed roofs, tried to memorize capitals, and snuck sips of gasoline behind the garages of Cedar Falls most of his life.*

Dear Young Iowan:

You are a honyock from some windswept plain, and we all come from nowhere in particular. This notion should give you all the humility needed to approach the world with respect and tolerance. Look this world in the eyes, and shake its hand, squeeze it firmly. The world will respond with joy because it loves the black dirt from which we all come, to which we all return. Be a person of quality, and the devil will never call collect. Remember the specific gravity of the light in each morning as you walk to school, climb playgrounds, or run through ditches chasing butterflies. Remember looking into the sloughs and woods in April to see that first green haze of spring buds.

We honyocks do leave to see wondrous sights out in the world. The restless pollen of adventure has sprinkled down upon us from the rafters and eaves of every barn, home, AMVETS hall, church, convenience store, and fire station since we arrived here. Maybe some other place will lure you away with its charms, its people, its tongue, but you will carry this place with you like a wistful lover wondering what might have been. You will always be welcome in a land that seduces with its seasons, simplicity, and subtlety. Remember the low, slow fireworks of lightning bugs. Remember the smell of different weeds when you spike them with a tree spade or root them out in a garden.

Some might ask a honyock about potatoes, Cincinnati, and corn. Remind them of *The Music Man,* and the West Bend Grotto, and try not to bring up why there are two concession stands at the Field of Dreams. Some out there will dismiss this place as "the fly-over," they might hum "Dueling Banjos," or speak of cultural desolation—never defend this place. Some folks forget

Genesis and that everywhere is technically "God's country." Artesian wells of pessimism, distrust, and hatred are found everywhere; try not to drink the water. Only in quantity can the devil dance and be happy. Remember the sweet earthy smell of blue-ribbon livestock mingling with the smell of cooking donuts and the taste of cotton candy at every fair. Remember those days when the first dry air of winter rides a warm afternoon breeze and blushes trees the fierce colors of mighty warriors.

Read every book you can under your blanket with a flashlight, study a globe, learn a few words in another language, and play a few simple songs. Ask your family about their lives, make as many friends as you can, jump off every shed roof that won't break your leg, swim naked in a creek or a pond, steal kisses down by the river, and take one small sip of gasoline when nobody is looking. Try to learn as many capitals as you can remember, and ask adults *why* until they chase you from the room. You'll need these things, little honyock; it's all on the test. Remember somebody once called that half-decayed corncrib their castle, starship, clubhouse, or hideout and left sandwich crumbs for the raccoons to find at night. Remember the quiet air of a fresh snowfall and how wood smoke can somehow connect you back generations to wherever it is that we came from.

Most of all, look this world in the eyes, and squeeze its hand when you shake it.

Sincerely,

Ron

Sharon and Tom Savage

Sharon and Tom Savage met as students at Iowa Wesleyan College in Mount Pleasant, Iowa, and went on to obtain Master's degrees from the University of Iowa: Sharon's in social work and Tom's in college student personnel. Both have recently "retired"—Sharon from a career as a therapist and child abuse worker; Tom from twenty-six years as a counselor at the local community college. Sharon Savage continues to be an adjunct faculty member at the local community college, a licensed independent social worker and a member of the National Association of Social Workers.

The Savages are both heavily invested in their home community of Muscatine: both maintain memberships in the Greater Downtown Muscatine Association, the League of Women Voters, and Writers on the Avenue. Sharon's outreach includes membership in the Iowa Foreign Policy Leadership Council, among others, as well as active involvement in statewide elections. Tom's eclectic activities center on books and literacy, including membership on the Muscatine Friends of the Library Board and independent work as a writer of Iowa history—work which has resulted in a forthcoming book on Iowa place names. The Savages have two sons, a daughter-in-law, and a granddaughter. They are proud owners of Muscatine Books and More and part owners of an Iowa Century Farm.

Dear Young Iowan:

Books work well in barns and on tractors. They fill the spaces made open by our fields and farms. Through books, our Iowa world can be made as varied and exciting as the cities and with all the richness and depth of our quiet purpose, our soil. Our minds are formed by the books that we experience as young adults: Tom, for instance, grew up in a southeastern Iowa farm home filled with practical reference books—atlases, encyclopedias and the like—as well as page-turners written by Nathaniel Hawthorne, Charles Dickens, Edgar Rice Burroughs, Jules Verne and many others; Sharon remembers treasuring, in particular, the copy of *Angels Came Down* given her by her Sunday school teacher, and, of course, *Grimm's Fairy Tales*.

Given how much we loved books growing up, it's no surprise, looking back on it now, that we envisioned a bookstore. Four years ago we were lucky enough to plant that dream in a storied, 1845 building that had been a drugstore and hardware store for most of its life in downtown Muscatine. Its ten feet high tin ceilings, punctuated with skylights, throw a lovely light off the oak floors, to our shelves filled with books, and back again. Our store occupies a street where flags fly for the Fourth and along which our town parades. It seemed like the center of the community to us and the center is where we wanted to be!

To begin with, we bought a stock of books that we thought might interest our friends and neighbors and, naturally, ourselves. We found that every acquisition we made came from an inside-out knowledge of particular folks. We bought history books for the many Muscatine history buffs we know. We bought books that reflected our own educational backgrounds in the social sciences and education. And, since the birth of our granddaughter, we've been filling out the children's section. The bookstore seems to have grown with us at every stage. We expected ours would be a quiet little mom and pop (grandma and grandpa in our case). Instead, we have experienced a life journey.

We found that an independent bookstore is defined by, and reflects, the community. Every town has resources and people that deserve notice; our bookstore has given some of those people and organizations in Muscatine a forum. We have benefited more from saying yes to the plans and ideas of others than by any insight or planning of our own. Our role has been primarily to unlock the door.

Our shop also gives us the opportunity and privilege of meeting you. We can pour you a cup of coffee, show you the pictures of our granddaughter. We can tell you what good books we have read lately and also give you an idea, minus names, of what the local ministers, or teachers, or doctors, or politicians are reading. We can learn about your interests and hopes and dreams. We can help you find just what you are looking for.

Ideas, all kinds, distinguish a bookstore from other businesses. Our products are thoughts, beliefs, viewpoints. That's why a bookstore becomes a natural location for discussion, exploration, and learning. The message to you, young Iowan, is not necessarily to go forth and open an independent bookstore, but this: find a location where you are free to express yourself; find people with whom you can exchange thoughts and dreams. Let those people be the kind who will respect your efforts at the "big answers" while still appreciating your love of the smallest details.

No matter where you are in Iowa—or America, for that matter—a logical first place to look for visionary folks is in the local bookstore. We learn from each other. This is what an independent bookstore is all about.

Yours in the stacks,

Tom and Sharon

Robert Sayre

An emeritus professor of English at the University of Iowa, Robert Sayre is a longtime resident of Iowa City and an advocate for Iowa and for its prairies, a purpose that led him to author Take This Exit: Rediscovering the Iowa Landscape *and* Recovering Prairie *as well as to a former position on the advisory board of the Aldo Leopold Center for Sustainable Agriculture. As a scholar, Sayre is a leading authority on American autobiographical writing and the author of* The Examined Self: Benjamin Franklin, Henry Adams, Henry James *and* Thoreau and the American Indians.

Dear Young Henry Wallace:

Brilliant, enterprising, industrious, and independent-minded young Henry Wallace! Still in your teens, you became skeptical of Iowa farmers' traditional ways of selecting their seed corn. Every fall they took the best looking ears, dried them, and used the biggest kernels for the next spring's planting. What could have been more logical? It was also heartily endorsed by the experts and extension agents, who rode around the state on a "Seed Corn Gospel Train" preaching to farmers on precisely how to do it. But, young Henry Wallace, you took such seed, planted it behind your father's house in Des Moines, planted other rows with little rejected kernels, and showed that there was no difference in the final product! You proved the seed corn gospel mere voodoo.

So you became interested in research being done in the East on the cross-pollinization of corn. You studied at Ames with George Washington Carver, and since your grandfather had founded *Wallaces Farmer*, which your father and you, too, eventually edited, you were well positioned to know about and publicize this. Pollen from the tassels of one stalk could be taken and used to fertilize the silks of the ears on another stalk—something that naturally happens but could be controlled by selective detasseling and pollinating. Corn seed could thus be bred "hybrid" to develop specific desirable traits.

The further study and perfection of the process would take years. All through the 1920s and 1930s you underwrote the research and development, principally through your Pioneer Hybrid Company. It also took years to

Good Sense from the Good Folks of Iowa

215

convince farmers of the advantages of planting hybrid seed. They had to buy it, and buy it new every year, for the kernels in hybrid corn, having been pollinated from their own and similar tassels, would only produce genetic freaks. But Pioneer's salesmen and your energetic allies like Roswell Garst of Coon Rapids had other forces on their side.

During the Depression, when you were Secretary of Agriculture, you attempted to reduce corn production (and thus raise prices) by paying farmers to reduce the number of acres they planted, which they did. But by planting those acres in hybrid corn, which was more productive, they could grow nearly as much or more than they grew before. So your government programs indirectly encouraged planting hybrid seed—and the growth of your company.

Hybrid corn, in being developed to be more uniform in height and to have stronger roots and stalks, could also be more efficiently harvested. No longer did farmers and their families and hired men need to walk down the rows, picking by hand. It could be picked by machine, which became a great advantage during World War II, when farm labor left to fight and work in factories. The old pastures and hay fields were then not needed for horses and could also be planted in corn. By the end of the War, nearly all the corn in Iowa would be hybrid.

Finally, hybrids could be developed that resisted pests, survived droughts, and were tailored to different fertilizers, soils, and growing seasons. It became possible to plant corn year after year, in the same field, just applying more and more nitrogen fertilizers—"continuous corn."

Such were the blessings of hybrid corn: greater productivity, less labor, and greater reliability. A farmer who did not accept such blessings, Garst said, was a sinner! He even invited Nikita Khrushchev, in the midst of the Cold War, to come to Coon Rapids and witness these hybrid miracles. Khrushchev did, and went home to tell Russia's collective farms to try to repeat them.

But the curses of your work, Henry, have also been many.

Hybrid corn has made farmers more dependent, for they now have to buy their seed and the fertilizers and pesticides, which means borrowing money each spring to put in their corn crop. The genetic variety of seed corn has been lost. Planting so much corn impairs the soil. The nitrogen fertilizers that run off into rivers have now produced a "dead zone" of oxygen-depleted water in the Gulf of Mexico that is the size of New Jersey, while the pesticides have poisoned both rivers and ground water.

Beyond these environmental damages, our overabundance of corn is itself a curse. It has depressed prices and narrowed farmers' margins of profit, forcing them to try to "get big or get out." Cheap corn has led to everyone's looking for more ways to use it—feeding it to cattle, which is bad for their digestion, and using it to make corn syrups and sweeteners, which are making us overweight. Also, to reduce corn surpluses, our government subsidizes its export to countries like Mexico, where it puts their farmers out of work.

The specialization and mechanization that go with hybrid corn have also been curses. As farms have grown larger, rural population has fallen, undermining the schools, culture, and economies of country towns. Iowa today has scarcely more people than when you were growing up, although the United States is now four times bigger. The Iowa of tomorrow may look as empty as the Great Plains.

Monocultures are dangerous. Sugar cane was for centuries the curse of Cuba and the Caribbean Islands. "King Cotton" impoverished the land and people of our South. And King Corn is doing the same to Iowa and the Middle West. King Corn's new partners are the confinement operations that crowd thousands of hogs into long, putrid buildings and produce gigantic "lagoons" of excrement, further fouling our air and water and landscape.

And believe it or not, Henry, the curses of corn may soon be even worse. Ethanol—automotive fuel made from corn—is providing yet another use for it. Many people promote this, saying it means new jobs and helps reduce oil imports and will raise corn prices. But unless very carefully controlled, it surely means just more of all these abuses—more fertilizers, more pesticides, still bigger farms, and more rural decay. To grow more corn (when we should be growing less), farmers will plant it again on hilly land, which will erode and renew the kinds of problems you later tried, as Secretary of Agriculture, to correct during the Depression.

You never foresaw all this when you undertook to disprove the Seed Corn Gospel. Nor are you alone to blame for it. Still, it is a troubling legacy for you to have left us. The influence of your work on hybrid corn now seems far greater than the influence of your work as Secretary of Agriculture, Vice-President, and candidate in 1948 for President, when you led your failed campaign against Harry Truman for peace with Russia. You were the emblematic Iowan—optimistic, generous, hard-working, scientific, and independent. You wanted to help farmers become more wealthy and productive and help the human race to have more food. But I have heard it said that had the same amount of research been applied to seed corn that was later applied to hybrid corn, it too might have been improved, and with fewer negative consequences. The person who said this was none other than Norman Borlaug—your spiritual heir.

What I hope is that somewhere in Iowa today other brilliant young persons are at work on new projects that will reduce our state's dependence on corn and lead to a more diverse, profitable, and less destructive agriculture.

Sincerely,

Robert F. Sayre

James Calvin Schaap

Jim Schaap has been teaching literature and writing at Dordt College in Sioux Center for thirty years. He has authored the novels Romey's Place, In the Silence There Are Ghosts, *and* The Secrets of Barneveld Calvary, *among others. Schaap's novel* Touches the Sky *and his most recent work,* Startling Joy: Seven Magical Stories of Christmas *earned an Award of Merit from* Christianity Today. *Among Schaap's other books is a collection of short fiction,* Paternity, *stories about fathers and their children, and* Fifty-Five and Counting: Essays and Stories.

Dear Young Iowan:

You won't understand all of this now, but someday I hope you will.

Here's the story. Once, when your mother was a little girl, she and her brother and your grandparents were on vacation somewhere around Lake Michigan. We were driving along on a country road tunneled by beautiful pines and hardwoods, somewhere amid those sprawling woods of the Great Lakes region where I grew up, a forest of green.

Your grandma reached for my hand. "How long are we going to be here?" she said.

When people are married for a while, they learn to hear more than words. In a flash I knew your grandma was, well, antsy. "What's the problem?" I said.

She shrugged her shoulders. "I don't know—I feel weird," she told me.

At that moment, I realized I'd become an Iowan—not because I was feeling what your grandma was, but because I knew exactly what it was she felt.

Claustrophobic. We Dutch Iowans have a word for it, one of the few Dutch words I know. The word is *benauwd*, and it means, in a way, "painfully locked in"—no wiggle room, as if the world were an MRI tube. Lots of people feel it on elevators or in small places too full of people. There's a little nausea in it, something of an upset stomach. With those huge trees on both sides of the road, your grandma felt hemmed in, almost sick. She was *benauwd*.

Good Sense from the Good Folks of Iowa

And that's because, as an Iowan—and a northwest Iowan particularly, I think—she was born and reared keeping an eye out west where the weather comes from, watching whatever it is that's coming down the pike. In the forest, she could see nothing but trees.

That people joke about the weather out here—you've heard them, I'm sure—doesn't mean they don't take weather seriously. Your great-grandpa, home from World War II and just starting a family and a farm, spent two long years working as a mechanic in town just to help him cover the loss when a hailstorm wiped out his very first crop. Hail insurance doesn't stop folks from watching the sky today as closely as your great-grandpa did. I do. So does your grandma. She always has.

We've got a big sky here, a big and beautiful sky. Honestly, if you take the time to look, it's just about the most incredible canvas you can imagine, God Almighty the only real master artist. Out here where you live, the most incredible light show gets staged with almost every dawn and dusk. If, as the Psalmist says, "the heavens declare his glory," then the Creator's splendor is almost declared quite unceasingly before us. I like that.

It took me awhile to see all that myself, to hear it, even to listen. And it will take you a while, too, I'm sure. But this vast open space you live in now: it'll find its way into you, just as it did Willa Cather and Frederick Manfred and a ton of other prairie writers. And as it has your grandma—and even me, born and reared five hundred miles away on Lake Michigan.

Out here in the northwest reaches of the state of Iowa, we're in a land that's the opposite of *benauwd*, nothing at all like an MRI tube. All that wide-open prairie and its crowning glory the heavens are forever on display—so much to see you can't help live in the kind of humility that comes easily by way of the jaw-dropping silence of sheer awe.

Someday soon you'll be a teenager. You'll look around and tell yourself that in this place where you live there is no happening stuff. You'll say there's nothing here.

But sometime, later on in your life, out here on the emerald edge of the Great Plains, I hope you'll come to know, as your grandma and I do, that so much nothing all around is really, really something wonderful.

Love,

Grandpa

Nancy Schmidt

Nancy Schmidt grew up on a farm near West Chester in Washington County. She attended Mid-Prairie Community Schools and went on to Iowa State University and a subsequent career as a home economics teacher in Janesville, Wisconsin for eleven years.

Schmidt, her husband Alan, and their children, Ryan and Lisa, returned to the family farm in Iowa when Schmidt's parents retired in 1981. They farmed for fourteen years and now rent out the family ground. Since 1984 Schmidt has worked for Iowa State University Extension as a county youth coordinator, a county director, and is currently an area youth field specialist working out of the Keokuk office.

Dear Young Iowan:

We Iowans who grew up prior to Roundup Ready seeds experienced cutting the volunteer corn out of the beanfields and so became experts in commiseration. The routine included getting up early in the morning to get a few hours of work completed before the hot, humid day set in, taking a jug of ice-cold water along, and making sure the bean hook or corn knife was sharpened. There was always lots of complaining about this unpleasant chore, but misery loves company, so working with a small group of other kids made things more bearable.

Then there were the days of mulching the garden. As soon as the vegetables were up and the garden was weed-free with the help of a rototiller and good old-fashioned hoe, it would be time to mulch the garden, especially the tomato patch. Invariably, it would be the windiest day of the year when one of you would be putting the newspaper down, and the other would try to shake the straw on it before the wind blew the newspaper across the field. Again, there was lots of complaining about this troublesome chore, but the ripe, juicy tomatoes, along with the variety of other vegetables produced in the garden, somehow made it worth the trouble.

As summer turned into fall, stoking the wood stove provided lots of adventure as well. The Sunday afternoon trips into the timber to gather wood provided a great family outing. While Dad cut and split wood, we kids

Good Sense from the Good Folks of Iowa

helped load it on the wagon or sled and carried it to the pick-up. You know how the old saying goes: "He who cuts his own wood is twice warmed." But we knew better: He who cuts his own wood is warmed about five times—cut, split and load; unload to the wood pile; carry from the woodpile to the house; enjoy the warm wood heat; carry out the ashes.

So how did these tasks help us as we grew up in Iowa and how can they help you? They helped us develop our work ethic, which Iowans are noted for and something employers universally desire. It helped us learn about how things grow and about the tender loving care it takes to produce those growing things. It gave us an appreciation for the food supply that is so readily available to us. It made us thankful for a warm shelter over our heads. We learned responsibility and knew that we were needed as an important member of the family.

These are things that we learned through our experiences growing up on an Iowa farm that we now pass on to you, our children. And hopefully you will be able to provide similar experiences to your children, helping them to learn important life lessons.

Sincerely,

A Caring Mom

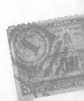

Susan Troutman See

Susan Troutman See grew up in northeast Missouri, but has now lived in her adopted and beloved state of Iowa longer than she lived in her birth state. She is a piano instructor at Iowa Mennonite School and has a teaching studio in her home as well. Susan See and her husband Richard reside in Washington. They are the parents of two grown children, Nathan and Rachel, and one retired greyhound named Andy.

Dear Young Iowan:

> *The wolf will live with the lamb, the leopard will lie down with the goat, the calf and the lion and the yearling together, and a little child will lead them.—Isaiah 11:6*

As you know, I was born a fighting Welsh Presbyterian. Our little church boasted a large American flag in the front of the sanctuary. In the foyer, a plaque on the wall named all the soldiers from the area who had fought in the wars of the twentieth century. The lesson I learned was that war is horrible, but sometimes necessary. Countless times I was reminded by my parents that I had not lived during World War II, and so I could not understand what I did not know.

I am now almost fifty-two-years-old, well into the second half of my life. Living near a Mennonite community in Iowa for the past twenty years and teaching piano at a Mennonite high school have changed me and the way I view many things. Although you, your brother, and your father have always supported me in my rather recent decision to become a Mennonite, I wanted to explain to you more fully why I could put it off no longer.

Day after day of teaching at this little school set on the scenic Iowa prairie, I witness a way of living that is too consistent to be labeled an aberration. Here, I continue to also be a student of the Mennonite way of life.

Over the years, the gentleness of those involved in this school has proven more powerful than any sermon I have ever heard. You see, Mennonites believe that violence is wrong, and they live out this belief even when it is unpopular. The "Sermon on the Mount" found in *Matthew*, Chapters 5-7, is about God's kingdom on earth right now, not a kingdom saved for some future generation and time.

Since September 11, 2001, it is a little more difficult to be a Mennonite. People question your "patriotism" and your unwillingness to support a war. Recently, the Iowa Girls Athletic Association informed the Mennonites that their school would not be allowed to hold regional volleyball tournaments in their home gymnasium. Even though they qualified for the honor with their winning record, the school does not play the national anthem prior to games, and according to the State Association, that constitutes good reason for moving the games elsewhere.

But Mennonites are about so much more than just being labeled "conscientious objectors." Being a part of a historic peace church, along with the Quakers and Church of the Brethren, means praying for your enemies. It means asking God's blessing on the whole world, not just America. It means working for peace and justice in nonviolent ways. It means taking the words of Jesus as the truth, not just to be used when convenient, but in how we live each day.

Mennonites have been persecuted for their belief in adult baptism and their pacifism for over five hundred years. The story of Dirk Willems in 1569 stands out as an example of one who was faithful unto death. Willems had been imprisoned near Asperen, Holland, because of his Anabaptist faith. He managed after a few weeks to escape. It was winter time and the river was slightly frozen. The assistant jailer chased the prisoner across the ice and fell through. Dirk Willems had to decide whether to keep running to safety, or turn back and save the dying man while the other jailers looked on, unwilling to risk their own lives to save the man in distress. He pulled his pursuer to dry ground. Immediately the jail bailiff ordered the freezing but now-saved junior officer to arrest Willems. It is reported that he did so after some hesitation. Willems was imprisoned once again, and later he was burned at the stake. I can think of no warrior who was more courageous than this man who certainly knew what his fate would be for "loving his enemy."

Mennonites are neither Catholic nor Protestant. They have a "third way." They suffer with Christ as his disciples and refuse to inflict suffering on others through violent ways. The weapons at their disposal are those of the spiritual sort.

Evil must always be resisted. Being a pacifist does not mean being passive. It does mean to find ways other than torture and killing to implement change. Violence breeds violence, while ways of peace, if given a chance to work, allow for great miracles to happen. There are countless real life examples over the centuries that prove this to be true.

When I was your age, I was freshly out of college, feeling like I had it all. I was starting my chosen career and was eager to spend time with my new husband. I was a little too young to give much thought to Vietnam. I was too far removed from the scenes of the civil rights movement to care, and too insulated from the problems of the world to ask questions.

But I would challenge you, young Iowan, to search for the truth now instead of waiting a half century. Search for truth in society, in government, and most of all, in your spiritual life. God has given me the Mennonite Church as a vehicle to help me find inner peace and to work for peace on this earth. Even so, I do not believe that it is mandatory to be a member of a "peace church" to be peaceful. Bloom where you are planted. Read lots of books, continue to study the Bible fervently, do not accept authority without question, look for diversity, act boldly, "get in the way," and find a passion for loving even your enemies.

If you hold to my teaching, you are really my disciples. Then you will know the truth, and the truth will set you free.—John 8: 31-32

With a love that knows no bounds,

Mom

Good Sense from the Good Folks of Iowa

Daniel H. Smith

Daniel H. Smith assumed the post of executive director of School Administrators of Iowa in July 2006 after serving as superintendent of the Cedar Falls Community School District for sixteen years and, before that, as superintendent of the Knoxville and Dunkerton school districts.

Smith's first administrative position was as high school principal for the Manning Community School District. His career in education began as a middle school teacher. He received his Bachelor's degree in secondary education from Dana College in Blair, Nebraska, his Master's degree in secondary education from The University of Nebraska at Omaha, and a doctorate in educational administration from The University of Iowa. Smith's commitment to education extends beyond the classroom to involvement in Junior Achievement, Rotary International, Chamber of Commerce, and the United Way, among many other good causes.

Dear Young Iowan:

Iowa is a small and caring state where a friend made today will most likely be someone you will encounter later in life. As a result, everything you do is "for the record." This is a good thing to know because it allows you to build your record purposefully and establish networks of Iowans who support you in our state and across the nation. This network also allows you to reciprocate, to support other Iowans when they need it.

This support begins in schools, neighborhoods, and churches. It is a part of the activities and sports teams we get involved in as we grow up here. It exists on the campuses of our colleges and other post-secondary institutions, and it continues in Iowa's places of work and worship, as we become adults.

What is so special about the kind of lifelong support Iowa offers? In particular, treating a person well today bears fruit long into the future. It allows you to take risks, knowing that friends outnumber strangers, friends that help pick you up if you stumble and that will join you in your success. It means that a young Iowan can look forward to being asked, "What part

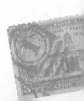

of the state are you from?" and "Do you know _____, who is also from your hometown?"

Most importantly, it means a friend is always just around the corner.

Sincerely,

Daniel H. Smith

Tracy Steil

After graduating from high school, Tracy Steil enlisted in the Army National Guard and subsequently served her country hauling bombs, mail, food, and other equipment in Saudi Arabia during Desert Storm. During the war, she met her husband Jerry, an Iowa native. Steil earned a BA in elementary education, a degree she puts to use daily as the county youth coordinator in the Humboldt office of the Iowa State University Extension Service. Jerry and Tracy Steil and their three boys live on a twenty-acre farm nestled among a few rolling hills near Livermore.

Dear Young Iowan:

Young people in Iowa today need to learn one thing: love.

The little boy peeks around the doorway when he hears his parents in the next room whispering to each other. When he looks into the room, mother is holding her husband's hand. The husband kisses her as he catches movement and sees the little boy is watching.

He says, "Brandon, come here."

The four-year-old runs across the room to join the couple. Dad picks him up, puts him between them, and they both give him a hug.

When we teach our young children to love, everything else important in life will follow.

Love,

Tracy Steil

Larry Stone

Larry Stone reports that he never outgrew his boyhood fascination with playing in creeks and exploring woodlots on the Warren County farm where he grew up. After a twenty-five-year career as outdoor writer/photographer for the Des Moines Register, *he now is a freelance nature writer and photographer. Stone has written four books, and his works have been published in a number of conservation magazines. He and his wife Margaret manage woodlands and prairies on their farm along the Turkey River near Elkader. They have two grown children and two grandsons who love to play in the dirt.*

Dear Young Iowan:

Maybe you don't need much advice, since you already seem to have a pretty good grasp of the essentials. You're inquisitive and curious—just as young explorers should be.

Don't ever lose that amazement—at the gooey feel of pond mud between your toes, the hypnotic sound of tree frogs *prrrring* at dusk, the tantalizing smell of wild plum blossoms, the sweet-tart taste of fresh tomatoes, the grace and beauty of a turkey vulture soaring among those cottony clouds, the flicker of fireflies dancing in the dark.

You're very lucky to be growing up in an Iowa that still gives you the opportunity to experience those sensory pleasures, and to have an extended family to help you discover joys of throwing rocks into a river, or watching a farmer bale hay, or sleeping out in a tent on a clear night when the coyotes howl and the full moon shines like a beacon over the fertile hills and fields and woods.

You know instinctively what some of us oldsters may have forgotten: the bumblebees and toads and rabbits and bluebirds and ants and snails and oaks and milkweeds and butterflies are just as much a part of this world—this community—as we are. Even now you worry that these other creatures, your friends, need a home—a place to feel as safe and secure as you do when you're snuggled in. For now, it's enough to accept those simple truths.

Good Sense from the Good Folks of Iowa

But as you grow older, I hope that you'll keep asking those penetrating questions, and that you won't accept simple answers to your queries.

No, maybe it's not okay to bulldoze a woodland or a farm field for yet another mall or automobile dealership. No, it's not enough to save a tiny, fenced-in, postage stamp of a token park.

Yes, kids and critters require open space to stretch their wings and their souls. Yes, you do want to be able to play in the creek, or go fishing, or run through a field of coneflowers and big bluestem. And our spirits need the renewal we find in plain old solitude—a place where you don't have to listen to growling engines, or smell a factory farm, or even see an artificial light.

Don't be bashful: speak up for those rights! And keep asking *Why?*

Love,

Papa

Rod Sullivan

Rod Sullivan grew up on a farm east of Sutliff that has now been in his family over one hundred and fifty years. He attended school in Lisbon, K-12, before moving to Iowa City in 1984 to attend the University of Iowa, where he received his BA in 1988. Sullivan continues to live in Iowa City with his wife Dr. Melissa Fath, a research scientist at the University of Iowa, and their three children, Rachel, Jordan, and BJ, as well as an occasional foster child. Sullivan worked in human services for several years before being elected to the Johnson County Board of Supervisors in 2004.

Dear Young Iowan:

Even though we have lived in town your whole life, you have seen what the farm can do to me. I get emotional. It is difficult to explain, and it strikes the city-bred as silliness. You always seemed to ask the most questions, so I have decided to attempt to give you the most answers.

"Where are you from?" To place-based Iowans, this question even precedes the ubiquitous, "What do you do for a living?" The way in which you respond to this question says a lot. For you, the answer may be easy. You can simply reply, "Iowa City." For me, the answer would be right in the center of Pioneer Township, far western section of Cedar County.

Most people will listen to my description, take a moment, then offer, "So what is that near?"

At this point, the conversation can take several twists and turns. My suggestion? Find out where the questioner is from.

Back when I was a Cub Scout, our tiny pack attended a huge jamboree in Galena, Illinois. There we met scouts from a French-speaking area of West Africa. We couldn't speak any French, and they couldn't speak much English. I think we parted ways with them thinking we were from Chicago. Funny thing is, they could have said they were from Chicago, and we would not have known the difference. Chicago—Africa—they are both quite a ways from Cedar County.

Good Sense from the Good Folks of Iowa

If the questioner is not a native Iowan, use bigger cities as your landmarks. "Roughly halfway between Cedar Rapids and Davenport," should do the trick. If not, just try "eastern Iowa."

If the questioner is a native Iowan, things can get interesting. You may be met with something like, "Is that near Lowden?" or " I know some folks from Bennett."

If the person is a fellow Cedar County native, it really gets fun. The conversation may boil down to, "Well, where are you at from the Ferguson place?"

"Everett Ferguson's or Dave Ferguson's?!"

Sometimes the conversation would go, "I went K-12 in Lisbon." This would usually be followed by, "Ah, so you are from a small town." Town? Town was miles away! Most days, I would have given anything to be in town!

We lived, it seemed, *way* out in the country. It was several miles to the nearest paved road. When Iowa expanded from three area codes to five, there was tremendous public concern over where the lines would be drawn. Public officials assured Iowans that the lines would be "in the middle of nowhere" so as not to affect customers. They put the line right between my mom's and my grandmother's, even though they live less than half a mile away from each other on the same gravel road.

So, when you first went out to the farm when you were just a little boy and innocently asked, "Where are all the peoples?" you were right on target. It is isolated. And it takes a certain mindset to deal with the isolation. Much of the romanticism I now feel for rural Cedar County was missing when I was a teen. I wanted rock and roll, not rock roads.

Now, Cedar County has lost many of its jobs. Most of the residents commute to Cedar Rapids, Iowa City, Davenport, and Muscatine. The jobs are alright, but not what they used to be. Most people live with an uneasy feeling that their job could be headed to Mexico, or China, or India—somewhere far away. Cedar County schools have met with the same fate—some elementaries are closed, and small town schools have consolidated. The families with young children did not go as far away as the jobs, but they, too, have gone. Things change, and not always for the better. Huge farms have replaced small farms. Machines have replaced men. When I was a kid, most of us lived in the country. Not so anymore.

Lots of people have moved away from Cedar County. This includes me. I left to attend the University of Iowa in neighboring Johnson County. I look around twenty-some years later and realize I have now put down roots in Iowa City. My children, I say, are *from* Iowa City.

I can rationalize with the best of them—the farm is only half an hour away. I still take my kids back to the farm a lot. For their part, I think they have grown to appreciate it. They like to visit their granny, and they sincerely enjoy the stories told back there.

Yet a part of me has always felt guilty. I think of my family, and it pains me to write this, but I never wanted to farm. Farming was always too lonely for me. I always longed to be in town, where it seemed there was a perpetual sandlot baseball game.

Farming itself seemed to be accompanied by an underlying pessimism. Even if those of us raised on farms were excited about something, we were always advised to temper those expectations. A soaking rain is met with comments like, "Where was this three weeks ago?" and "Too bad it won't last." The celebration of a big win by the local team quickly devolves into, "Next week is gonna take a much better effort."

Mom, Dad … we're going to have a baby. "That's wonderful, honey! Do you want a boy or girl?" *We don't care—so long as it's healthy.* I don't think those of us reared in rural Iowa lack hope; in fact, it is very much the opposite. Planting a crop in the spring requires a certain degree of optimism. It is inherently risk-taking. If we had no hope, farming wouldn't work.

Rather than expressing high hopes, rural Iowans have learned that it is better to keep those hopes to themselves. Expressing more than cautious optimism is seen by the neighbors as cocky and unwise. The lesson is that you are much better off being pleasantly surprised than dealing with a big disappointment. Rural people may not be simple people, but they are supposed to appear so.

Pessimism was not unique to my family. A neighbor friend grew up in a big family with a gruff father. When Iowa first instituted a state lottery, his family was sitting around the table, dreaming about the ways they would spend any winnings. The father would have none of such a foolish discussion.

He was a hard worker, who did not expect to get anything he had not earned. When pressed as to how he would spend these hypothetical lottery winnings, he replied, "I'd probably get a new engine for our old Fairmont." Simple man, simple plan.

My grandfather was, in some ways, a simple man. He wore overalls pretty much every day of his life. He told me more than once "Don't trust anyone wearing a tie." He didn't really mean it. I think. I was never quite sure. There was a twinkle in his eye when he said things like that. I wish all of the next generation, the great-grandchildren, would have had the opportunity to see more twinkle, and less of an old man ravaged by Alzheimer's. He was a very fine man. The kind of stereotypical person we Iowans are supposed to be, even though he is pretty much the only one I ever met.

I go back through the last paragraph and wonder aloud if I should use the word *simple* in describing my grandfather. Grampy knew a lot about almost everything. There wasn't much he couldn't do. I remember someone asking him for directions. These were the days before rural addresses; everything was simply Rural Route One. Grampy said, "Then head west about a mile and three-tenths, and go south. You'll run right into it."

I reset my odometer, and drive the same route. I crest the hill, see the destination. My odometer rolls over to 1.3 miles as I reach the drive.

Like my grandfather, I see myself as a complex person. I can be erudite in some ways, simple in others. One of my favorite, old-fashioned Iowa pleasures was peeing outside. I love peeing outside. As kids, we used to walk past the bathroom and out the door just to pee outside. Is it somehow better? Well, the kids who lived in town weren't allowed to do it. As country kids, we needed to play up any and all advantages, no matter how dubious. Dust is still my enemy, even though I have lived in Iowa City for years. I still worry about the amount of precipitation we get, no matter how easily I can water my tomatoes. It is an old saying, but it rings true: you can take the boy out of the country, but you can't take the country out of the boy.

Love,

Rod

Mary Swander

Mary Swander is the author of numerous books, including the latest, The Desert Pilgrim: En Route to Mysticism and Miracles. *Swander received her MFA from the University of Iowa and is a Distinguished Professor of English at Iowa State University. Her ancestors homesteaded in Carroll County, and she now lives in Ames and Kalona.*

Dear Young Iowan:

I'm driving down Highway 22 from my home in rural Kalona, Iowa, site of the largest Amish settlement west of the Mississippi River, toward Riverside, site of the largest casino in the state. The storefronts in Riverside, a once lovely downtown nestled on the banks of the English River, are boarded up with rotting lumber nailed across their once-graceful, red brick facades. Even the antique store has gone out of business. The most upscale establishment on the block is Murphy's Bar and Grill. But Murphy's and most of the other businesses in town, it seems, are gambling on gambling to make them more prosperous.

We need to place our bets. We can continue to support casinos, hog confinement and slaughter houses in the state of Iowa, or we can provide sustainable, family-centered jobs that encourage a healthy environment. We can lay our money down on more stinking air, lost farms, and lost fingers, or we can embrace the new agriculture. My generation has begun a change. We've stopped chasing our losses and have returned to the simple idea of growing, selling, and consuming our own food within our own borders. We've led the way with pesticide-, hormone- and drug-free products. But we can't continue this journey on our own. We need young Iowans to travel with us.

When the die settles, the promised ice cream store may open its doors in Riverside, and the little old ladies will have their night out slipping their social security checks into the jaws of the slot machines. But what about the bigger picture? Why does Iowa have more gambling per capita than any other state in the union? And why did casinos, factory farms, and meat

Good Sense from the Good Folks of Iowa

packing plants become Iowa's idea of "economic development?" How did we get into such desperate straits?

Once, Iowa had been a prosperous agricultural state made up of a web of small family farms, small towns and medium-sized cities. Then agribusiness, largely supported by the U.S. subsidies, forced out small family farmers who in turn supported the merchants in the small towns. Wal-Mart and other box stores put a tighter squeeze on the local hardware, clothing, and grocery stores. Then in the 1980s, high interest rates pitched scores of wobbling small farmers into bankruptcy. A rural suicide prevention hotline was established for the first time.

Young people who received excellent educations in our school systems took one look at the boarded up storefronts, polluted lakes and streams, and moved away. "So how are we going to keep those young Iowans down on the farm?" we asked ourselves. During the Farm Crisis, the state started to try to address its dying downtowns and brain drain with craps and caged pigs. Since that time we've lacked the imagination to come up with a better plan.

The roulette wheel spins around and around and while it mesmerizes most, others have sought their fortunes away from the cigarette smoke, blaring music and lights. In quiet pockets of the state, sustainable agriculture has taken root. Small organic farms, CSAs (Community Supported Agriculture), the Iowa State University Leopold Center, the Women, Food, and Agriculture Network, the Slow Food Movement, the Amish, food co-ops, restaurants, farmers' markets, and a host of other groups have joined forces to create an alternative economy, one based on the old-fashioned Iowa values of self-reliance, entrepreneurship, and wholesome, local food. The movement has gained such momentum that even Wal-Mart is trying to cash in on the trend and will soon stock its shelves with "organic" junk food.

The choice is yours right now. Take a first step. Buy local, natural or organic food. Okay, okay, I hear you protest that healthy food is too expensive.

Here are some tips.

Eat at home—Or bring a bag lunch. You'll be amazed how much money you'll save when you stop slapping it down for those giant-sized hamburgers and soft drinks.

Join a CSA—That's a farm that sells shares of their yields. You pay a seasonal fee, and, in return, you receive an abundance of fruits and vegetables—often delivered right to your door. The produce is fresh, reasonably priced, and eliminates the middle person. You can often volunteer at the farm and pick your own.

Buy local produce at your own farmers' market—Make it a social occasion and meet new friends. Hear some live music (many markets feature local talent). Take in the sensations of the colors, shapes, and textures of an array of fruits and vegetables that you've never tried.

Own your own pig—Throw out your ice cream and fill your freezer compartment with meat purchased directly from an individual farmer. You'll be amazed how this transaction will cut costs for you. At the same time it will support family farmers who create a good life for their livestock.

Join the movement—and cultivate a vegetable plot in your backyard or in a community garden. Tend some chickens. Grow tomatoes in a pot on your balcony. Grow sprouts on your windowsill. Commit yourself to one small bit of rich Iowa soil and rediscover what made this state what it is.

All right, so now your head is out of the smoky casino and under a wide-brimmed straw hat. Now you're wondering where to begin with your grocery bag full of winter onions, asparagus, lettuce and spinach. What do you do with these things? Cooking from scratch can be overwhelming for someone who has spent a lifetime heating up processed food in the microwave. Get on your cell phone and call your grandparents. Ask them for a couple of simple recipes. They'll be thrilled to hear from you and happy to help. Go to the library and spend a half hour paging through cookbooks. Go online and look for fast, easy recipes that can become your standards.

Ah, but doesn't this all take time? Yes. But less time than all those trips to the convenience store. Less time than all those trips to the dentist filling your teeth from all those sugar-filled treats. Less time than all those trips to the doctor treating obesity, diabetes, cancer and a host of diseases linked to poor diet. Insulin shots. Chemo and radiation. Now those things take time. Once you join the movement, you'll also have more food on hand. You'll reach in the freezer for hamburger or step out in your garden to pick a ripe zucchini. You'll feel better. Your mind will be more alert. You'll have a better appreciation for the natural world.

Good Sense from the Good Folks of Iowa

I'm turning around on Hwy 22 and heading back toward Kalona where the downtown businesses are open, well-kept, and adorned with pots of blooming red geraniums on the sidewalk. I'm heading back to Kalona where a local organic dairy, a local produce auction house, and numerous farmers' markets are helping to fuel the economy. I'm driving past plots overflowing with broccoli, cabbage, bush beans, beets, and carrots, ringed with beautiful red cannas and purple petunias. My stakes are garden posts holding up fences full of scarlet runner bean blossoms, hummingbirds fluttering around the bright red petals. I'm heading back to Kalona and picking up hitchhikers. Want a ride?

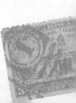

Sarah S. Uthoff

Sarah S. Uthoff works as a reference librarian at Kirkwood Community College in Cedar Rapids. A lifelong Iowan, Sarah and her family have lived in Johnson County for six generations. She received both her history education BA and her Master's of library science from the University of Iowa. An active researcher, Uthoff's main interest areas include Laura Ingalls Wilder, one-room schools, and historic foodways. She has been published in several professional magazines and spoken at numerous regional and national conferences. Uthoff currently lives on the family farm, where they raise Hereford cows, Suffolk sheep, chickens, and a large garden.

Dear Laura Ingalls Wilder:

I have been fascinated by you ever since I was read your Little House™ books by my grandparents when I was a very little girl. Not only was I lucky enough to grow up in the heart of the Midwest, near all the places you lived, but in Iowa, which has three strong Laura connections of its own. Not only did you live in Burr Oak, but your sister Mary went to the Blind School here at Vinton and your papers are housed at the Herbert Hoover Presidential Library at West Branch.

Laura, wanting to know more about your times led me to study history and eventually to teach it. Wanting to know more about how you lived led me to get involved with living history, where I learned some of the same skills that you and your family used every day: how to cook on a wood cookstove, how to use a treadle sewing-machine, and how to gather eggs. The more I found out about you the more I wanted to share with others through my research writing and presentations. I put my first presentation about you together as a 4-Her when I was in the fourth grade, and I'm still going strong!

I keep an image of you, Laura Ingalls Wilder, in my heart, and when I am faced with a problem, I think of you and all the challenges you faced—from grasshopper plagues, to house burnings, to the death of your newborn son. I think of how you prevailed to have a beautiful farm and to write such wonderful books that have touched so many lives. I think of the times you

Good Sense from the Good Folks of Iowa

were afraid and how you overcame that fear—how some everyday thing would frighten you and you would face it anyway, resolved.

I most remember your words, "It is still best to be honest and truthful; to make the most of what we have; to be happy with simple pleasures and to be cheerful and have courage when things go wrong." I try to apply those words in living a life that would make you proud. I hope young Iowans will follow the example of your many faithful readers and take up the challenge of living an honest, resilient life.

Admiringly,

Sarah S. Uthoff

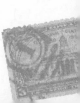

Christie Vilsack

As First Lady of Iowa, Christie Vilsack worked to build a sense of community among Iowans by promoting family literacy, public libraries, school libraries, and computer literacy. Through her literacy foundation, Iowa Stories 2000, she created a process that helped seventy Iowa communities inventory literacy programs and helped groups whose literacy needs were not being met. Each year she raised resources to give every Iowa kindergartener a book about Iowa by an Iowa author, and she has traveled to over four hundred and fifty Iowa libraries urging Iowans to support public libraries.

As a result of thirty years of experience working with middle school, high school, and college students, Christie Vilsack has a special interest in issues concerning adolescents. She speaks to high school students about opportunities in Iowa's new economy as well as the changing nature of high schools and the value of higher education. The former First Lady is also a devoted mother of two sons: Jess, an attorney for Polk County, and Doug, a law student at the University of Colorado.

Dear Young Iowan:

When Tom was finishing law school and I was finishing my third year of teaching, we received a letter on yellow legal paper from my dad, a small town lawyer in Mount Pleasant, Iowa. At the time, we were living in upstate New York and considering establishing a law office there or in western Pennsylvania, where Tom had grown up.

My dad gave us so many good reasons for coming to Iowa we had to consider it as an option. As much as I loved Iowa, once I left, I never expected to come back. However, once we started making a list of all the advantages of Iowa, the list grew longer than both the New York list and Pennsylvania list. (One of my worries was that people in my hometown would always think of Tom Vilsack as Christie Bell's husband and that he'd never have an identity of his own. Now I laugh when I think of that fear.)

My dad was a wise man. He was right to say that in a small town we would be able to become leaders in the community quickly. He was right to say we could make a good living with Tom's salary as a small town trial lawyer and mine as a teacher. He was right that being near family was

Good Sense from the Good Folks of Iowa

important. He was right that a small town in Iowa is a great place to raise children.

For thirty years, we have enjoyed living in a small community in Iowa. We value that sense of community, and recently, in our travels around the country, we have heard people speak about a yearning to feel connected to other people, a desire to feel part of a community.

Some of the reasons for staying or returning to Iowa are the same now as they were then. Some of them are different.

Today you can still become a community leader quickly, especially if you choose to live in our county seat towns. You can also be part of building the new Iowa economy, an economy based on feeding, healing, and fueling the world.

With our ability to produce wealth from our soil on a yearly basis, we have the ability to move beyond feeding our crops to cattle and hogs. We have the opportunity to turn corn into 3,500 different projects, including medicines and vitamins, substitutes for plastic, and fashionable clothing. Our focus on value-added agriculture, laser and robotics technology, insurance, and advanced manufacturing means that we will be able to create jobs that pay the kinds of wages that attract more young people like you to Iowa.

In the past few years through our Vision Iowa program, we have been able to improve the quality of life in our small towns and major cities. We have concentrated on creating recreational and cultural opportunities for young singles and young families.

In small towns, you'll see new baseball diamonds, theaters, and fitness centers. In our cities, you'll see major event centers, museums, libraries, and river walks.

The changing landscape of Iowa is our welcome for new Iowans to come join us. We are becoming more diverse, more connected through high-speed Internet, and we've learned to balance work ethic with the ability to have fun, indoors and out.

We know that you may have been thinking of leaving Iowa. That's okay. I left, but I came back. I hope you will, too, and not just to visit.

I hope you'll find that our small cities have all the amenities, and, with a short commute, allow people to spend more time with family and friends. I hope you find the friendliest, most welcoming people in our small towns and our cities that feel like small towns. I hope you'll remember or rediscover our commitment to quality education for children and adults throughout their lives. I hope you'll appreciate our commitment to community can-do spirit and our progressive attitudes about issues such as making our state the renewable fuels capital of the United States of America.

Our fields are full of opportunity. Our small towns and cities are beckoning. We hope that you'll stay or come home someday to the best place in the country to live, work, raise a family, and have a good time.

Sincerely,

Christie Vilsack

Timothy Walch

Timothy Walch has been the director of the Herbert Hoover Presidential Library Museum since 1993. He also serves as a trustee of the State Historical Society of Iowa. Educated at the University of Notre Dame and Northwestern University, Dr. Walch is the author or editor of sixteen books of American history including Uncommon Americans: The Lives and Legacies of Herbert and Lou Henry Hoover.

A Letter to Herbert Hoover, Future President, November 12, 1885

Dear Bertie:

As you leave for Oregon, I hope that you will cherish your memories of Iowa. You were born here and lived here at a very special time, a time when we carved this rich prairie land into farms and communities. I hope that you never forget us, and I pray that you will come back to see how we change Iowa and how Iowa changes us.

Life here can be harsh. You're only eleven years old but already you understand the meaning of heartache. Your father passed away almost five years ago and your mother died less than two years ago. There's no one here to care for you permanently, so today you go west to live with your Uncle John.

Although you'll be many miles away, never forget that you carry a bit of Iowa in your heart and on the sole of your right foot! I'll never forget the day that you were helping your father in his blacksmith shop and you stepped on a hot chip of iron. You were a brave little fellow, but I'm quite sure that the wound hurt a lot. Both your parents comforted you, so that scar will always be a reminder of their love.

I know that you don't have much to take with you to Oregon. In fact, everything you own fits into a small alligator-skin satchel that once belonged to your father. I heard that your grandmother sewed a couple of dimes into your coat pocket in case of an emergency. Spend the money wisely.

More important than material possessions, however, are memories. As the train takes you west, think about those wonderful times that you shared with your brother Tad here in West Branch. Together you explored the prairie with a real sense of adventure and arrived home everyday with a new fossil, a special stone, or an Indian artifact. The prairie was one big laboratory for the two of you.

And don't forget the fish the two of you caught in the Wapsinonoc Creek. There you were tempting crappies and lunkers to bite your precious night crawlers. Fishing taught you patience, and I never saw you give up until you had at least one fish!

There are so many other things that you should keep close to your heart as well: sliding down Cook's Hill after a fresh snowfall, earning money to buy firecrackers for the Fourth of July, enjoying band concerts and parades on Main Street, the smell and taste of Aunt Millie's pies, the gentle instruction from your favorite teacher, Mollie Brown. Life could be hard, but there was a lot of love as well.

Knowing your sense of adventure and self-reliance, I'm guessing that this journey west will be the first of many for you during a long and productive life. You've told me of your dream of going to college someday and becoming an engineer. Many of us here in Iowa believe that you will follow that dream.

Let me offer you a bit of advice about college. Whatever you do, hold fast to the friends you make in college. Whether you become successful or struggle through hard times, your college friends will stay true to you. In fact, I hope that you also will find a bride among those friends. You could do no better.

And after college, I hope that you will follow your instincts wherever they lead you. I believe the new century will belong to your generation. I expect that you and others like you will travel the earth and spread the word of our nation's ingenuity and ambition. If you do become an engineer, I am confident that you will be successful; perhaps you will become a man of wealth and influence. It's too soon to say that about a boy of eleven, but Bertie, I believe in you!

Given your abilities, Bertie, you might even achieve high office, perhaps even the Presidency of the United States. Wouldn't that be something?—a boy from Iowa becoming president! I know that it's only a dream, but it is the American dream.

I do, however, want to caution you about success. Your parents taught you about your responsibilities to others in need. Should you have the ability and the opportunity to feed, clothe, and shelter those less fortunate than you, I trust that you will do so. This would please your mother more than anything else you might do with your life.

Whatever happens to you in life, don't let adversity sway you from the path of public service. Your mother taught you the Quaker way so you know well that we have all been put on this earth to serve. If you are knocked down in that quest, pick yourself up and begin anew. Never forget that the Lord will always be with you. Your mother understood this well and often spoke at Quaker meetings about the inner light. Her face beamed when she spoke of God and her sermons deeply moved all who heard her voice. At night, when you are tucked into bed and soon to go to sleep, listen for your mother's voice. She will guide you through this life to the next.

You have been well-prepared by scripture. Your mother insisted that you read a passage of the Bible every day, and you embraced the challenge, finishing the good book before your eleventh birthday. I asked you once if you had a favorite verse, and you quoted Proverbs: "Where there is no vision, the people perish; but he that keeps the law, happy is he." That's good advice for all of us.

I have great confidence in you and high expectations, young man. Long after I'm gone, I expect that you will be doing good things for millions of people. I also know that you won't care one lick about credit. You'll take satisfaction in a job well done—that's the Iowa way.

Remember us, Bertie, as you travel the world. Remember the rolling prairies, the rivers and streams, the small towns and communities. And most of all, remember the people. You will always have a home here in Iowa, dear Bertie.

Ed Williams

Ed Williams is a fifth-generation Iowa farmer who founded Century Farm Harvest Heat in 2002 to sell corn/pellet stoves. After farming for thirty years with his father and uncle near Iowa City, Ed now works "sun up to sun down" promoting a bioeconomy where plant-based material will be used for fuel, fiber, and chemicals. Williams served twelve years as a commissioner with the Johnson County Soil & Water Conservation District working on soil and water quality projects. Since 2003, he has been a director with the BIOWA Development Association as it coordinates the creation of Iowa's bioeconomy.

In 2005 Century Farm Harvest Heat established the George Washington Carver BioEconomy Award at the Johnson County Fair to encourage 4-H youth to investigate the possibility of new careers made possible by an agricultural renaissance. A book on the Century Farm Harvest Heat community entitled the feel-good heat: pioneers in corn and biomass energy *is forthcoming.*

Dear Young Iowan:

Since you first responded to my bioeconomy stump speeches with an exuberant "Mr. Williams, I'm a big fan of biomass!" I've learned so much from you. Now that you're about to embark on your first (of many I'm certain) research, collaboration, and book project, I thought it would be a chance to send you some words of observation, not necessarily wisdom.

Being born in Oelwein made you a native, but the twenty-five years since have truly made you an Iowan, now and always. I know you've expressed frustration with the lack of opportunities in your home state. One so educated, bright, and enthusiastic should be able to find worthy challenges suited to her talents. Still, you may need to travel before you return to contribute in your special way. As you temporarily make other states your home, you'll find yourself not only absorbing the views of the locals, but also imparting your own young wisdom, wit, and vision bred right here in the Heartland.

In your travels "abroad," get ready for the inevitable and unoriginal "Iowa jokes." Laugh politely, roll your eyes, and maybe even patronize them, for they know not what they do. You'll find the sophisticates on the coasts may

Good Sense from the Good Folks of Iowa

not differ much from those right here in your own backyard, Iowa City, the University of Iowa, the "Athens of the Midwest." Once, after politely listening to an anti-agriculture diatribe from one much more educated than I, I wondered about the correlation between education and ignorance. If it weren't so, why is this most educated, enlightened community we both love to call home so darn ignorant about so many things?

So take along your rural Iowa common-sense attitude, combine it with your education, passion and idealism, and spread it among those who will joke about Idaho and Ohio. I'm sure they'll be surprised by the real sophistication expressed by one so young.

Share with them the names of Borlaug, Van Allen, Vonnegut, and George Washington Carver. Some were not born here and others didn't stay long, but all spent time in this strange, appealing land we call home. Those who left all returned, if only for a visit. They all found unique talent, inspiration, and vision in their time spent in this "fly-over" state.

You and I both realize that the world is poised for a transformation not seen since the Industrial Revolution. Your "fan of biomass" statement the day we met showed your awareness of that. We've both expressed frustration that Iowa humbleness and rut-stuck thinking seem to ground us in our past rather than launch us into the future—a future where Iowa could truly be a beacon of this new economy.

Iowa is such a good state, but we could become a great state with just a little more bravado. Why this "we're not worthy" attitude seems to pervade the Iowa psyche is beyond me and must be left for others to study. Swati Dandekar once told me that Iowans need to brag more: "Don't think of it as bragging about yourself, but rather like bragging about the grandkids." Maybe that would be a good way to force us to step out of our comfort zone.

The mention of Swati brings to mind something else I think you'll find helpful in your travels and upon your return. Even though I have pride in Iowa talent, I think I've learned more, sometimes much more, from the "outsiders," those who have chosen to migrate here and remain. Whether it be Swati from India or Georg Anderl of Genencor via New York, these people truly see us Iowans for who we are and who we can become. Though they may not be "one of us," they truly love who we are. Their "outside looking in" approach must be listened to carefully.

Maybe your generation of Iowans, with your unmatched frequent flyer miles and globetrotting habits, will be the one to break the mold. Maybe you and those you've grown up with will be able look at Iowa with new eyes from a global perspective. You'll surely have the advantage of much more data, knowledge, and observations than I or your parents could ever have imagined. Please take that knowledge and turn it into wisdom.

I know not only you but many of your peers reluctantly leave the state. Hopefully a large share of you will be back, bringing with you this wisdom along with your enthusiasm for making Iowa and indeed the world a much better place.

In closing, may I please borrow from your oft-read closing to the many e-mails I've received from you—the one from Baba Dioum:

In the end we will conserve only what we love

We will love only what we understand

We will understand only what we are taught.

So, my dear young Iowan, I'm certain with your Iowa roots and world travels you will soon be able to "conserve," "love," "understand," and "teach" us all. We'll wait for your return and conserve this great good state in the meantime.

Kevin Woods

Born in Mount Vernon, Iowa, in 1955, Kevin Woods was raised on the same farm his grandfather brought his young bride to in 1926 and where, in his youth, Woods worked the same ground as his father and grandfather. When not working on the farm, Woods writes that he "squandered" a great, free education at Mount Vernon High School by becoming expert in "wrenches, girl-ogling, and cigarette smoking."

After serving in the Air Force in Idaho, Woods earned an Associate's degree at Des Moines Area Community College, which eventually led him to a position as staff engineer at the Square D Company in Cedar Rapids, where he has worked for the last eighteen years. Known for his sometimes contrarian, always engaging letters to the editor, Woods is married, with what he describes as "an assortment" of children, stepchildren, and grandchildren. He writes that Iowa is a "blessed place, mostly for what it hasn't got."

Dear Young Iowan:

The single concept you need to get your brain around to live successfully in Iowa or anywhere else is to stick with the Truth. The first rule of Truth is that you do not get something for nothing.

Your immediate reaction may be "No duh, geezer," and in that you might be justified. Many assume wisdom exists in gray heads, but the dirty little secret is that all we gray-hairs have done is managed to stay on the sunny side of the dirt longer than you have.

Real truth is more rare than you might think, and sometimes less gray. Isn't every media and cultural outlet you've been exposed to—TV, radio, print, Internet, movies—all telling you in one way or another that you can and should, and indeed deserve, to get any and all that your heart desires? From fitness to investment to romance, hasn't the theme generally been "no pain, all gain?" You should know this is BS. The idea is peddled by folks intent on manufacturing another compliant, enthusiastic, hyperconsuming generation—in short, a generation like mine.

Where did this mindset of "relative truth"—this something-for-nothing culture—start? I don't know exactly, but I think future social anthropologists will identify the gradual urbanization of America as the beginning of the culture of make-believe. Many of the lessons that refute the something-for-nothing mindset were learned on what used to be called "family farms." When I was born in 1955, Iowa was a place of such farms. By family farm, I mean a comparatively small, by today's standards, couple to several hundred acres farmed by an extended family. By extended family, I mean a collection of blood relatives who lived and worked intimately enough with each other to develop the love, dedication, tolerance, and oftentimes contempt of one another that are part and parcel of such family businesses.

Let me make clear I am not disparaging those making a living in industrial agriculture. They are intelligent businesspersons doing what any sensible businessperson would do, and that is dealing with what is. Farms have been getting fewer, bigger and more industrialized since at least the Industrial Revolution, so nothing new here. Undeniably these economies of scale have afforded much of the globe food of great quality and quantity, transporting many from famine to plenty. But the statistics do not speak to what has been sacrificed on the altar of agricultural efficiency and urbanization. As the separation of people from land becomes virtually total, my generation, the "Boomer Generation," The-Generation-That-Can't-Quite-Get-Over-Its-Bad-Self, has almost put the finishing touches on a culture of total make-believe, where all you have to do is make the minimum payment, where you can indeed get "something for nothing," and where there is no such thing as "too much," even when it is apparent to anyone paying attention that we are drowning in excess.

By contrast, if you are nose-to-nose with the care and tending of crops and livestock from the time you can walk, you can be a great dullard and absorb nature and farming's lessons of cause and effect. If you don't tend to your assigned chores, animals don't get fed, weeds flourish, and things die. Sometimes even with heroic effort, things still die. You see the unblinking reality of the seasons and their inability to acknowledge or accept excuses. The cycle of life, birth-to-death, will unfold before your eyes and somewhere along the way you will realize that you are not exempt from these processes any more than any other creature. You understand that there is quite a messy process getting meat from hoof to cellophane, a process you will not see in a Disney movie, or in the Mega-Mart under soft lights and Muzak.

It's easy to see the effects of the culture of something-for-nothing. It used to be, for example, that gambling was viewed for what it is, a moral and intellectual failing, a tax on the statistically challenged, in other words, a vice. It was relegated to the backrooms of taverns, where it was joyfully acknowledged as illegal, and sin, and therefore still fun. Now it has become a substitute for citizens taking responsibility for paying for services they want, ensuring the more pathetic of their brethren pay the tab. The greatest manifestation of the culture of something for nothing, and perhaps a fatal one, is our unwillingness as a nation to pay as we go even as our national debt hurtles towards nine trillion dollars. If no one has bothered to tell you yet, you will pay for my generation's party. We don't have the moral fortitude to pay for the services we want, so we just charged it to you and your children. We were hoping you wouldn't notice until after you picked out a nice rest home for us.

I guess I have arrived exactly where I didn't really want to land, young Iowan, at the end of a curmudgeonly rant. I suppose I could have said to you simply: seek truth wherever you find it and be honest enough with yourself to recognize it when you see it. If you can discipline yourself to see what *is* true, not what you *want* to be true, you will be miles ahead of many of your elders. But, much like keeping you out of the middle of the street, insisting you eat your vegetables, and sweating your safe arrival home after a night out—these countless acts of parental love and vigilance—it's always more complicated than a bumper sticker or greeting card can explain.

Still I say: stick with truth, and you'll do fine.

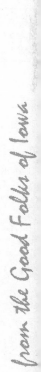

from the Good Folks of Iowa

About the Editor

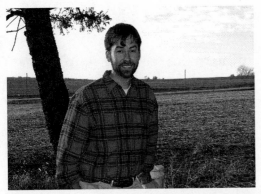

A graduate of Iowa City High School and an alum of Iowa State University, Zachary Michael Jack was raised on the Mechanicsville, Iowa Heritage Farm his family settled before the Civil War. Prior to his years as a college English professor, Jack served as a section editor for the *Tipton Conservative* and worked as a children's librarian and bookmobile driver at the Ames Public Library. He is the author of two Midwestern-centered books of poems—*The Inanity of Music and Wings* and *Perfectly Against the Sun*—and the editor of three collections of agricultural and conservation essays: *Black Earth and Ivory Tower: New American Essays from Farm and Classroom*, *The Furrow and Us: Essays on Soil and Sentiment*, and *Love of the Land: Essential Farm and Conservation Readings from an American Golden Age, 1880-1920*. *Black Earth and Ivory Tower* and *The Furrow and Us* have both been nominated for the Theodore Saloutos Memorial Award for the year's best book in agricultural history. Jack's international writing residencies have taken him to Ireland's Tyrone Guthrie Centre, Mexico's Great River Arts Institute, and New York's Blue Mountain Center. He teaches in the English Department at North Central College and is proud to call an Iowa farm his home.

Good Sense from the Good Folks of Iowa

About the photographers & cover artist

Ed Heffron (pgs. 206/207) was born and raised on a farm near Albia in south central Iowa. In 1969, he moved to Iowa City to complete a BA in journalism. In 1971, he began working as a medical photographer in the Medical Photography Unit at University of Iowa Hospitals and Clinics. He completed an MA in instructional design in 1976 while continuing to work. In 1986, Heffron began working as an ophthalmic photographer in the Department of Ophthalmology and remains in that position today.

Michael Harker (pgs 100/101) has been a professional photographer for over 35 years. He spent his first twenty-five years in advertising photography throughout the Midwest and the last ten years as an ophthalmic photographer at the University of Iowa Hospitals and Clinics.

In 1993 he began doing a documentary in B/W large format photography of Iowa barns, which led to the publication of *Harker's Barns: Visions of an American Icon* in 2003 and *Still Standing: A Postcard Book of Barn Photographs* in 2006, both by the University of Iowa Press. In 2008 they will publish his B/W monographs on Iowa's county courthouses and Iowa's one-room rural schools.

The photographs in this book represent his continuing growth as a documentary photographer of Iowa's architecture and rural heritage.

Mark Paul Petrick (pgs. 53/54) is an award-winning artist and photographer. His work in a variety of media, including photography, video, performance, printmaking and installation art, has been exhibited in prominent venues such as The San Francisco Museum of Modern Art, The Walker Art Center, The Art Institute of Chicago, and The Des Moines Art Center, among others. Over the last 15 years he has been working predominantly in black and white photography, with much of his work created in his home region of southeast Iowa for regular publication in the *Iowa Source* magazine.

Richard Sjolund (pgs. 129/130) was born in the Upper Peninsula of Michigan and grew up in Milwaukee, Wisconsin. He earned an undergraduate degree from the University of Wisconsin-Milwaukee. Dick then moved to California to work as a biologist for NASA on the Biosatellite Project and stayed in California to earn a PhD from the University of California-Davis. He joined the faculty of the Biological Sciences Department at The University of Iowa in 1968, and for 34 years he conducted research in the area of cell biology and taught courses in electron microscopy and human biology.

Photography has been his hobby since childhood and also played a major role in his research, especially in the production of images from light and electron microscopes. He taught photography to biology and medical students at Iowa and maintained a university darkroom. More than 15 years ago, he began to equip his microscopes with digital cameras, and he was an early adopter of digital image production using computers. He has retired from his faculty position to devote himself full-time to creating photographs. He now teaches classes in digital photography in conjunction with camera stores across the state of Iowa.

Rod Strampe (pgs. 151/152) was born in O'Brien County, Iowa in 1932 and currently resides in Iowa City. He studied at Morningside College and The University of Iowa and began working as a professional photographer in 1949. While a member of the Professional Photographers of America, he participated in juried national shows and was accepted to the National Permanent Loan Collection of the Professional Photographers of America. His most recent one-person exhibit was in Iowa City at Riverside Theater in the fall of 2006. Previous exhibits include the Old Post Office Gallery in Iowa City and the Sioux City Art Center. His images were published in connection with the 2003 Harvest Lecture, *Finding the Center of the World* at Old Brick in Iowa City.

Shelly Maxwell (cover artist) has lived in Wisconsin, Minnesota South Dakota, Illinois and Iowa—and brings these Midwestern states into her scrapbooking creations. She has been scrapbooking and card making since her youngest child, Charlie, was born in January, 2001. What started as a hobby is now part of who she is. She loves the textures, colors and creative outlet of scrapbooking and is currently employed at Reminisce, a scrapbook and design business in Coralville, Iowa, where she helps with retail and as a scrapbooking instructor.

Materials used on the cover layouts: Chatterbox violet dahlias and violet parlor roses used for background, authentic Iowa postage stamps adhered to Making Memories chipboard letters, Reminisce "Andria" paper, DCWV typewriter paper, Scotch transparencies, Heidi Swapp clock faces, Doodlebug paper posies, and miscellaneous paper flowers, brads, and foam dots.

Additional Ice Cube Press Books of Midwestern Interest

Firefly in the Night: A Son of the Middle West, Patrick Irelan
1-888160-20-9, $16.95
A candid and humorous story of a life repeatedly interrupted by emergencies. Irelan tells his story the only way he can, with more humor than the events recorded might seem to require. As a child he learned a set of values from his parents and other elders. He has lived his life according to those values, but with occasional revisions that have allowed him to survive the absurdities of modern times.

River East, River West: Iowa's Natural Borders
1-888160-24-1 , $12.95
Writings by David Hamilton, John Price, Gary Holthaus, Lisa Knopp, and Robert Wolf, with "creekography" by Ethan Hirsh, on the meanings, history, folklore, nature and ideas of the two rivers bordering our state. As this book shows, the Mississippi and Missouri Rivers are much more than the water that flows in them.

Prairie Weather
1-888160-17-9, $10
Iowa is at the crossroads of the elements—just above our heads whirl otherworldly tornadoes, and summers bring bone-drying droughts, while winter brings walls of snow. In our region of four seasons, we can learn much from our weather. Writing and photographs by Jim Heynen, Mary Swander, Deb Marquart, Amy Kolen, Ron Sandvik, Mark Petrick, Ethan Hirsh, Robert Sayre, Thomas Dean, Patrick Irelan, Michael Harker, Scott Cawelti, and a foreword by Denny Frary.

Living With Topsoil: Tending Our Land
1-888160-99-3, $9.95
A full-fledged exploration via Iowa's finest authors into living with our state's world-famous topsoil. New and valuable writing by Mary Swander, Connie Mutel, Michael Carey, Patrick Irelan, Thomas Dean, Larry Stone and Tim Fay, and an introduction by Steve Semken. Jose Ortega y Gassett once wrote, "Tell me where you live and I'll tell you who you are." You'll find out what it means to live in the land of amazing topsoil once you read this book.

Good Sense from the Good Folks of Iowa

The Good Earth: Three Poets of the Prairie
1-888160-09-8, $9.95
Surprisingly, there is a strong tradition of prairie poetry in Iowa. This work features the prairie-based works of legendary poets Paul Engle, James Hearst and William Stafford, examined, respectively, by Robert Dana, Denise Low and Scott Cawelti, with a foreword by Iowa farm poet Michael Carey. In the tradition of place-based stories, this book finds connections between spirit and place. As if that isn't amazing enough, this collection also includes one previously unpublished poem by Iowa's famed Writers' Workshop director Paul Engle.

Prairie Roots: Call of the Wild
1-888160-12-8, $10.95
An exploration into the meanings of the wild in the Midwest, featuring one of the last published essays of the late Minnesota author, Paul Gruchow. This intriguing collection explores other facets of Iowa and the prairie landscape: a fascinating examination of landscape art by Joni Kinsey, the results of the "grid" system laid upon our land by Robert Sayre, poetry by Mary Swander, the flight and call of geese by Thomas Dean and a discovery of giant worms by Steve Semken. Photography by Rev. Howard Vrankin.

Words of a Prairie Alchemist, Denise Low
(Poet Laureate, State of Kansas)
1-888160-18-7, $11.95
The Great Plains of the North American continent have dramatic seasons, intense colors, alchemical thunderstorms, and epic winters. Denise Low has emerged as one of the most trusted writers of this region. With a balance of drama and finesse, she describes the juncture between the natural world and the human realm of literature.

Ordering Information:
Books can be ordered directly from our web site at
www.icecubepress.com
or by mail (check/money order) by sending to
Ice Cube Press
205 N Front St.
North Liberty, Iowa 52317-9302

(shipping $1.50 first book, .25¢ each additional)

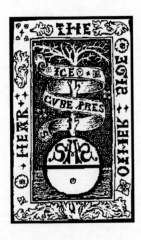

The Ice Cube Press began publishing in 1993 to
focus on how to best live with the natural world
and understand how people can best live together
in the community they inhabit. Since this time,
we've been recognized by a number of well-known
writers, including Gary Snyder, Gene Logsdon,
Wes Jackson, Annie Dillard, Kathleen Norris, and
Barry Lopez. We've published a number of well-
known authors as well, including Mary Swander,
Jim Heynen, Stephanie Mills, Bill McKibben, and
Paul Gruchow. Check out our books on our web
site, with booksellers, or at museum shops, then
discover why we are dedicated to "hearing the
other side."

Ice Cube Press
205 N Front Street
North Liberty, Iowa 52317-9302
p 319/626-2055 f 413/451-0223
steve@icecubepress.com
www.icecubepress.com

a bow to my partners
Fenna Marie & Laura Lee
and a grand right and left